D1109713

After

the Diagnosis

Transcending Chronic Illness

JULIAN SEIFTER, MD

WITH BETSY SEIFTER, PhD

Simon & Schuster

NEW YORK   LONDON   TORONTO   SYDNEY

Simon & Schuster
1230 Avenue of the Americas
New York, NY 10020

First Simon & Schuster hardcover edition August 2010.

SIMON & SCHUSTER and colophon are
registered trademarks of Simon & Schuster, Inc.

For information about special discounts for bulk purchases,
please contact Simon & Schuster Special Sales at 1-866-506-1949
or business@simonandschuster.com.

The Simon & Schuster Speakers Bureau
can bring authors to your live event.
For more information or to book an event,
contact the Simon & Schuster Speakers Bureau
at 1-866-248-3049 or visit our website
at www.simonspeakers.com.

Designed by Ruth Lee-Mui

Manufactured in the United States of America.

1   3   5   7   9   10   8   6   4   2

Library of Congress Cataloging-in-Publication Data
Seifter, Julian.
After the diagnosis : transcending chronic illness /
by Julian L. Seifter ; with Betsy W. Seifter.
p. cm.
1. Chronically ill—United States—Biography. 2. Chronic diseases—United States—
Biography. 3. People with disabilities—United States—Biography.
I. Seifter, Betsy. II. Title.
RC108.S445 2010
616'.04720922—dc22   2010007186

ISBN 978-1-4391-2304-1
ISBN 978-1-4391-3497-9 (ebook)

For Austin and Eleanor Weisberger, David Weintraub,
Sam and Eleanor Seifter, Andrew and Charlie

Contents

Introduction   1

1. Doctor-Patient 101   5
2. My Name Is Lucy Rooney   27
3. Too Sick. Not Sick. Just Sick Enough.   53
4. More Things in Heaven and Earth   79
5. Who Will I Be Today?   108
6. Going Fishing   132
7. Just My Luck   154
8. The Growing Point   179
9. Caretaking   201
   Conclusion: Bluefish   222

   Acknowledgments   233
   Bibliography   235
   Notes   237

After the Diagnosis

Introduction

My next-door neighbor Rick comes over to the fence that separates our houses and wishes me happy New Year. The Rick of the new year looks very different from the Rick of years past: he's gaunt and pale, and his hair has turned white. Still, he's recognizably himself—same tilt of the head, same long stride, same smile. From what I've seen of him lately, running his snowblower, stringing Christmas lights, rearranging things in his shipshape garage (which puts mine to shame), he's still the good householder he's always been. I'm not his doctor, but he's told me about his situation in bits and pieces, over the fence, so I've been following his story for a while. In middle age, Rick has been beset by a host of ailments, including diabetes. There are three of us with diabetes on the street, or three that I know of: not really all that surprising, given that 23.6 million Americans—7.8 percent of the population—have the disease.

Rick also has, or had, colon cancer, a rarer disease but with a higher risk of mortality. We never speak of mortality, though. Rick's conversation is always about what's just happened and what's going to happen next. His newest news is, he's finally had a colostomy. "I fought it. You know: 'the bag.' But now I'm feeling great."

I congratulate him.

Rick says, "Goes to show you."

I begin with something hard because this book is about hard things. It's tough living with an illness that's never going to go away. It's hard to live in a body that doesn't work right and to hold on to hope when the future's uncertain. But this book isn't only about the difficulties of being sick. It's also about the Ricks of this world, who find a way to live and thrive around, and through, illness.

Like Rick, my patients are gutsy and resilient. I want to give you their stories straight, without touch-ups, because it's the reality of their lives that will, I hope, strengthen and inspire you. But no story is completely "straight." One patient told me, "When you tell my story, don't let the facts get in the way of the truth." To get at a truth that is sometimes buried in details, I've changed some things, but my aim has always been to clarify and sharpen rather than blur or soften. I'm in the book too, pretty much unvarnished. I've made my share of mistakes in dealing with my diabetes, maybe more than my share. I'm coming clean here because I've lived long enough to face up to my errors and have even begun to do a little better. Maybe my wobbles will help you follow a steadier path.

As a way of organizing the many stories that follow, I've come up with a list of eight strategies for coping with a long illness. Here they are:

- **Be yourself.** Hold on to who you are despite the diagnosis.
- **Know yourself.** Find a balance between preoccupation and denial.
- **Transcend yourself.** Go beyond the physical to find sources of meaning.
- **Transform yourself.** Find and express unexplored parts of yourself.
- **Forget yourself.** Let go of obsession.
- **Forgive yourself.** Let go of remorse and guilt.
- **Grow.** Let yourself change over time.
- **Share.** Allow yourself to depend on others.

I've picked these phrases because they're brief and, I hope, memorable. The active voice has certain limits: "do this, do that" may be a good corrective for the passivity and helplessness that follow on the heels of illness, but I'm really after something deeper than "Just Do It." The most authentic growth depends not only on intention and effort but also on opening yourself to what has happened to you and letting experience change you. This more subtle process of transformation is at the heart of every story in this book. It's a transformation that, paradoxically, could not have come any other way: an illness that appears to close off possibility becomes, in the end, an avenue for creativity and enrichment.

The eight maxims I've listed refer to this process of creative change. You'll notice that *yourself* appears in all eight points. An assumption of this book is that the "self" is more various and flexible than people think. What we call our "identity" is really many different, and sometimes opposite, identities: contemplative and active, compulsive and dreamy, self-disciplined and self-indulgent. We need all of our selves to live our lives, particularly when we're faced with adversity. Successful living requires us to be, at different times, the person who follows rules and the one who thinks outside the box, the person who takes nothing on faith and the one who suspends disbelief.

After the Diagnosis tells the stories of people who found within themselves the means to transcend their bad luck. They did it by drawing on all aspects of themselves, as circumstances dictated. They were able to adapt, accommodate, change, revise, and, most of all, play. Being sick is serious business, yes, but that doesn't mean you have to clench your fists and grit your teeth. There's a concept from the ancient world, revived in the Renaissance, known as *serio ludere*—"to play seriously." *Serio ludere* was shorthand for a set of ideas on how to live: Contain opposites. Embrace variety. Hold two thoughts at once. Be rational and informed (*serio*) but also creative and joyful (*ludere*).

Chronic illness doesn't necessarily diminish life; it can actually enrich life by inviting us to access parts of ourselves that might otherwise lie hidden. The first story I tell is my own, both because I know it best and because it says something about the doctor-patient relationship. Standing at the intersection of those two roles, I've been able to look in both directions and to reflect on how that relationship can be most healing. So I begin with my residency training, a period that coincided with my getting sick. The succeeding chapters examine the eight strategies, focusing on patients who've done well despite their illness. I've changed their names but not the circumstances of their chronic conditions. I'm their doctor and have done my best to help them, but their stories have also helped me. I offer them here, in hopes that they'll do the same for you.

1

Doctor-Patient 101

I'm sitting in a darkened ward next to the bed of a man in distress. He's in his sixties, though he looks much older, with a lined face and salt-and-pepper hair; his chart says he has heart failure. He's sitting propped up on pillows, his face blue under the fluorescent light. His breath comes unevenly, and he struggles to get words out. He is Italian, he tells me. I nod. He's been a cabdriver his whole life. He's driven the streets of New York; the map is up here, he says, pointing to his head. He's driven some important people around the city; Mayor Lindsay, one time. I nod. He gulps for air; his lungs sound wet. He has a little garden on the roof of his apartment building, I should see his tomatoes. I nod.

His breath grows raspier. He looks at me. I hold his hand. A shudder runs through him, his eyes close, he slumps forward. His body is still.

It's my first night as an intern, 11:00 p.m. I pronounce him dead.

I began my internship terrified, the way everybody does. Moving from paper cases to real ones, from role-playing to responsibility, is a giant step. Add to that the fact that I was doing my house staff training at Jacobi Hospital—the "Jake"—a medical center in the Bronx where residents were basically it from the get-go: draw the bloods (and run them to the lab), perform the spinal taps, man the crash cart, insert the central lines into the neck or groin. A hospital for poor people, understaffed and underfunded, expected its trainees to do a lot of the heavy lifting. My first night on, I called my wife at midnight. I'd already seen a cardiac arrest, a lung collapse, a platelet crisis. These people were sick. These people were dying.

I said, "Pack the bags and meet me outside in ten minutes. We're leaving town."

I stayed. In the course of the year, I earned my doctor stripes. Mostly I loved it. But I had a secret. Somewhere around the beginning of my internship, the house staff was sitting around the Metabolic Unit testing patients for Wilson's disease, Addison's disease, Crigler-Najjar syndrome (an enzyme defect that causes jaundice and affects the brain). The diseases were interesting, but the tests were insanely boring.

I said, "I have an idea: why don't we all do GTTs on each other?" A GTT was a glucose tolerance test. I'm still not sure why I thought of it, though maybe it had something to do with a question that had dogged me since childhood about unpleasant sensations I had after meals, after exercise, and sometimes in the middle of the night, when I'd wake up in a sweat. Was there something the matter with me?

Everyone agreed GTTs would be fun, so we drew bloods, recorded a baseline, drank cola, and took bloods every thirty minutes for three hours. By the end of ninety minutes, my blood sugar was over 200, which is a diagnostic sign of diabetes. Later I went to a friend to have my fasting glucose measured, and he told me it was "borderline." I decided to ignore it.

I'm the intern of the group, rounding with the team, walking down the hall discussing the last patient we've seen, when Phil, my resident, suddenly collapses. He's yelling obscenities, knocking over glassware. Then he's on the floor, writhing, arching his back, foaming at the mouth. The rest of us swing into action. Someone finds a tongue depressor to put between his teeth, and we're trying to get his blood pressure when someone says, "Give him glucose." It turns out that Phil is an insulin-dependent diabetic. He's in insulin shock: his blood sugar is plummeting, his brain is deprived of vital glucose. First seizure, then coma, then death. Severe hypoglycemia is what put the heiress and socialite Sonny von Bulow into a vegetative state for the rest of her life.

We put in the intravenous line and Phil revives instantly; his eyes fly open, his color returns. I'm not insulin dependent, I'm "borderline," but I know I don't want this to happen to me, ever. Of all the lessons I'm learning in my house staff training, this is the most visceral, the most personal. You don't want to cross the line and become the patient.

Inevitably, doctors and patients look at each other across a great divide. It's the chasm that separates the well from the ill, only wider and deeper. Most of the doctors I know, including myself, have an ambivalent relationship to sickness. On the one hand, we're drawn to it: we want to understand what goes wrong, we want to make it right, we want to save lives, we want to heal. On the other hand, disease is a source of dread and fear. Being a doctor is, in a sense, a way to underscore that "I'm OK, you're not OK." Sickness is not us, it's other people. In my years on the admissions committee at Harvard Medical School, I read numerous applicant essays that described growing up with an ill or dying family member. The personal brush with disease is often the driving force in the choice of medicine as a career, but it can be a double-edged sword. There's pain (and sometimes revulsion) in the past, somewhere. Donning a white coat may represent, in part, a wish to keep safe: I'm OK, even if you're not.

As I embarked on my own training, I felt ambivalent about illness. My father was sick. Life-threatening rheumatic fever when he was a child, treated with megadoses of aspirin, led to a life-threatening perforated stomach ulcer when he was in his thirties, and I was four. He had hypoglycemia, vitamin B_{12} deficiency, cysts on his kidneys, rheumatoid arthritis, and, later on, atherosclerosis and Parkinson's disease. He was a productive scientist who became chairman of his department; he wrote many papers, taught medical students, traveled widely. But within the family, there was a steady drumbeat of worry: Was he okay? Was he angry? Had he eaten? Had he slept?

Growing up, it wasn't enough for me to be simply healthy. I was superathletic, fit, strong: captain of the high school track team, tight end on the football team. The funny sensation I got after meets and games? I decided to ignore it. And when it came time to choose a career, my path was clear. I didn't want to be sick, that was for sure. I'd rather be the doctor.

The resident says to me, "The FUO? Mr. Bernstein? Go take blood cultures and get some sputum."

I'm the intern, the "new guy" who only recently learned what FUO

means: fever of unknown origin. I am also the body-products guy. Blood?
Sputum? Coming right up.

Mr. Bernstein is an old man with gray hair, pale skin, a paunch. I in-
troduce myself and apologize for disturbing him in the middle of the night.
He's barely awake. I massage the inside of his elbow, find a vein, stick in
the needle. Dark purple blood fills the vial.

"Sorry, I'll need some sputum, too," I say.

I ask Mr. Bernstein to cough, but he can't. I swab the back of his throat
to get him to deliver some sputum. No go.

I report back to the resident, who instructs me to bang on Mr. Bern-
stein's chest.

"I'm sorry, Mr. Bernstein, but I'm going to have to bang on your chest."
I bang. No go.

The resident comes with me the third time. Turns out it's the other Mr.
Bernstein, two beds down, who has the FUO.

One thing about being house staff: it's hard to form a relationship
with patients. You say hi, you make a little small talk, and then it's
mostly procedures. You're dealing with acute stuff, not the chronic
day in and day out. Also: you're young, and the people in the beds
are mostly old. The divide between the doctor and patient is perhaps widest at this point in an MD's career.[1] There's a whole lingo
that goes along with this sense of separateness: patients who are elderly, have unfixable ailments, or are suspected of hypochondria are
called GOMERs (as in Get Out of My Emergency Room); patients
with multisystem disease are described as having PPP, Piss-Poor
Protoplasm; children with pervasive developmental disorder are
FLK (Funny-Looking Kids). A patient who dies shortly after being
brought up from the emergency room is a QC, Quick Cool.

The worst phrase of all was SPOS—Subhuman Piece of Shit—which was applied to hopeless cases, the ones who'd come in just to die. (My fellow intern, watching two alcoholics stagger across the ER threshold, said, "Oh, look, a SPOS de deux.") Such jargon is (to say the least) crass, callous, politically incorrect, and our chief cautioned us never to use any of these phrases in front of students. These days there's a code of ethics governing doctor-patient relationships, plus a mentoring system to help trainees deal with the stresses of internship and residency, so there's much less trash talk on the wards. Back in the 1970s, such talk didn't accurately reflect how any of us felt about individuals we cared for. It was more a black humor tactic for dealing with the unremitting tensions and demands of the job. We fended off. We developed a thick hide. We expressed our exhaustion, hostility, and fear by using insiders' acronyms. We looked at patients as "them," not us.

There were always exceptions, people we got to know who dented our armor. I remember taking care of Slapsie Maxie Rosenbloom, an old-time Jewish boxer from the 1930s, and a celebrity in his day. He looked, at first glance, like just another GOMER—heart failure, pneumonia, cognitive confusion—but then we got to talking. He told me he was down on his luck: he'd gambled away all of his winnings, and things had been pretty disappointing since he left the ring. He had a cauliflower ear, a bulbous nose, gnarled hands. He'd worked for a while in Hollywood, cast as a gang member in crime movies; they told him he had the face for it. Slapsie and I got along great.

You could say that I felt "empathy" for Slapsie, though, really, it just felt like we were having a good time. Now we teach empathy in medical school in a series of courses called Patient-Doctor.[2] Whoever heard of teaching empathy? You either have it or you don't. But it's a complicated matter, less either-or than both-and. You can have genuine feelings for a sick person and still need a thick skin to deal with the onslaught of difficult cases and painful outcomes that are part of the house staff years.

We saw plenty of painful outcomes. At Jacobi, we got very sick patients, and many of them died on our watch. The ER rotation was particularly gruesome. I remember a mentally retarded kid who'd been wandering on Bruckner Boulevard and was hit by a car: he bled to death through his nose while the interns stood and watched. There was nothing to be done. I remember a man whose car had exploded when he was rear-ended on the highway. He was already dead when they wheeled him in, arms and legs in the air, blackened into a cast-iron mold of himself, smelling like charred meat. Nothing to be done.

It was beyond horrific sometimes. When I became a resident, one of my duties was to sign off on the DOAs—dead on arrivals—who came in by ambulance. There was the time I went out to meet the stretcher, and the kid lying there—twenty years old, a heroin addict, eyes fixed and dilated—was warm when I touched him.

Another night I went out to meet a DOA, and the paramedic waved me off. "Just sign," he said. "You don't want to see this." I explained that I actually did have to see the body; it was a requirement. He shook his head, took me into the ambulance, uncovered the body. The face was like nothing I'd ever seen, a pumpkin head, featureless; no eyes, no ears, no nose, no mouth. Turned out he was a college kid who'd been missing the whole winter; his body had been fished out of the river. I never heard the full story about the kid—suicide? foul play? I was just the resident; we never heard the personal histories. But I had nightmares about him for months afterward.

The smell of death, the look of death, became familiar. But we all had an itch to do something about it. We were the antideath squad. I remember when, as a student, I rotated through a gynecology clinic, and a woman who'd just undergone a D and C—dilation and curettage—was explaining the procedure to the next woman in line. The second woman, pointing to me, said, "What does he do?" The first woman said, "Oh, he watches." But watching wasn't good enough. One rule I'd learned from a stint in the merchant marine aboard a cargo ship: don't have your hands in your pockets. Make yourself useful.

I learned to do carotid sinus massage, jamming my fingers into the neck of a patient with cardiac arrhythmia. The first time I saw it, the procedure looked like attempted murder. I learned to thread tubes up people's noses and down into their stomachs; to plunge a thick-gauge needle between the vertebrae into the spinal fluid or stab through the skin into the chest; to slip catheters into urethras or jugular veins. As a student, I, who hated the sight of blood, stuck my hands into abdominal cavities, sewed up stab wounds, held retractors during operations. One time I brought in my landlord's finger (along with the landlord); he'd sliced it off cutting fish. The surgeon told us to wait a minute because he was operating on his dog in the ER.

I used to stare out the window, waiting for the sun to come up: sunrise meant I was finally safe from another admission, another crisis, another procedure. I worried all the time, especially when a patient died. Had I done something? Had I *not* done something? Better to have not done something, I thought. A physician friend of mine once had four admissions in a row, three of whom died that night. Had he done something? Had he not done something?

Everyone around us was dying or in danger of dying. My house staff training is, in my mind, bracketed by two occasions. On July 4,

1975, four days into my internship, I was walking home from my shift, and I kept stopping to scold fathers who were setting off fire-crackers with their young kids. I'd just come from a scene of carnage in the hospital—severed digits everywhere from backfiring Roman candles—and I couldn't believe the risks these people were taking. On June 30, 1978, I had completed three years of training, the third as chief resident, and was packing up for a fellowship at Yale–New Haven Hospital. I was sitting at Yankee Stadium on a hot, bright afternoon, looking at fifty thousand screaming fans, and it was surreal: how could all these people be well? Weren't some of them going to keel over any minute? And me without my cardiac paddles!

For three years I'd been living in a world of the very ill, and I'd learned to do something about death. On one memorable occasion in the emergency room, a man brought to the hospital with seizures was flatline—basically dead—for significant periods, requiring applications of CPR to jump-start his heart. When he woke up briefly, during one of his moments of sinus rhythm, I explained that I was about to insert a pacemaker, and he said to me, "I don't want to be resuscitated." I was chief resident by then, the ultimate authority in the ER at three o'clock in the morning, and I just went ahead and passed a wire into his heart, restoring a regular heartbeat. The next day, I visited him in his hospital room. He didn't mention the previous night; he just said, "Thanks, Doc." I told my team he'd been hypoxic: his oxygen-deprived brain didn't know what it was saying.

Through three years of taking care of sick people, I was never, ever sick. Never missed a day, never fell down on the job, never dropped a stitch. I was far away from being the person in the bed (and far from being Phil the diabetic, thrashing on the floor). I was at the top of my game. All the house staff had a hotshot air, stethoscope in one pocket, reflex hammer in the other. Our uniforms, like Superman's cape or a cowboy's holster, made us feel powerful. Despite the physical and emotional toll, we were having a strange kind of fun in those years. It was, at least some of the time, like playing doctor.

There was the game of Can You Get the Autopsy? Families usually felt that an autopsy was a violation; they didn't want their loved one to be cut open like a slab of meat. We made the usual pleas to persuade families to agree—"This knowledge will help other sick people"—but in private, we made up outrageous stories, things like: "We left a golden ball inside Mr. Smith's abdomen when we sewed him up."

There was the game of Instant Epitaph. A Russian Jew pronounced on the dead body of a Ukrainian who'd been in the tsar's army: "This is one dead Cossack."

There was the game of Tweak the Attending. Some attending physicians weren't too thrilled to round with us, because their outpatient practices suffered when they had to put in academic time at the teaching hospital. There was one doctor in particular whom we called "Shifting Dullness" (which has to do with ascites, an accumulation of fluid in the abdomen associated with cirrhosis of the liver; when you tap on a cirrhotic's distended belly to determine the degree of retention, the percussion is dull, and it shifts). It wasn't just that Shifting Dullness was bored with us; he was extremely boring himself. I needed some clinical gem to liven things up, so I presented him with a case of porphyria, a genetic disease that induces madness. (King George III of England had it.) As I was energetically describing the acute abdominal crises, the psychoses, the interesting chemistries, Shifting Dullness woke up. "Let's go see him!" he said enthusiastically. We were halfway down the hall to the patient's room when I was forced to confess there was no patient; I'd made the whole thing up.

There was *The Gong Show* (though perhaps you had to have been there), a TV talent show in which panelists expressed their displeasure by beating on a gong. I happened to own a mini-gong, from my travels in the Far East on a cargo ship, and I brought it to hospital rounds the year I was chief resident. When interns presented cases, it was gong—you flunk!—or no gong—good job! We were kids, basically, with the playfulness of kids, so to us this was hysterically funny.

While we were getting a workout emotionally, and exercising our senses of humors whenever possible, we were also flexing our brains. On the one hand, we were confronting life-or-death situations; on the other, we were engaged in mental tasks of a much cooler order: doing puzzles, solving problems, soaking up the wisdom of our elders, learning our trade.

Medicine is, in essence, a very long—perhaps never-ending—apprenticeship. My chief mentor at the Jake was Milford Fulop, tall (or tall to me, in the same way that Willie Mays was ten feet tall) and bespectacled, with a high domed forehead full of brilliant thoughts. His delivery was wry, dry, laconic. He didn't walk the halls, he prowled them, sniffing out cases that would teach us something. Milford liked basic medicine, a boon for us novices. He'd skip the exotic presentations, the VIPomas (vasoactive intestinal peptide-secreting tumors), the pheochromocytomas (adrenaline-producing tumors), and go first to the nursing home patients.

I remember visiting a bedside with him to talk to an elderly Jewish woman from the Bronx who had strange electrolyte abnormalities for no discernible reason. She also had a rash all over her body. I'd gone over her chart ten times, looking for a drug that might be the culprit, but she wasn't on anything that would cause a rash. I confessed to Milford that I couldn't find the cause, and he said, "Let's go see her."

He sat down next to her, took her hand, peered at her over the rims of his glasses, raised his eyebrows.

"Constipated?"

"Oh yes, Doctor," she said, "it's been just terrible."

He raised his eyebrows higher, as though to ask the next question.

"I've been taking ex-lax."

He turned to me, raised his eyebrows higher yet. *Voilà!* The laxative use, or overuse, had led to the disturbances in her blood and urine, as well as the mysterious rash.

To me it was magic. At the time, I thought I'd never be able to do that: take one look at the lab values and the symptom, run through the differential diagnosis at the speed of lightning, ask a one-word question, and arrive at a solution. This is called a heuristic: a mental shortcut arrived at almost without thought because experience has forged the connections so deeply. In his book *How Doctors Think*, Dr. Jerome Groopman makes the point that heuristics can lead a doctor astray—we need to stay alert to the oddball diagnosis, the array of alternatives. We need to think outside the box. But as interns, we were just learning the box. There's a saying in medicine: when you hear hoofbeats, think horses, not zebras. In other words, don't go for the exotic possibility, because it's far more likely to be the usual suspect. We were just getting the hang of what the usual suspects were.

Though most of our patients turned out to have garden-variety ailments, once in a while a zebra would appear. An illegal immigrant from South America came to the ER with a sore on his arm that turned out to be leprosy—a treatable condition, despite the popular mythology. The dermatology resident should have referred to it as Hansen's disease, the medical term for it, because the minute the patient heard the word *leprosy,* he disappeared from the ER, never to be seen again.

Then there were the rare findings that had nothing to do with diagnosis. At the old Lincoln Hospital, the Lords, a Puerto Rican gang from the South Bronx, burst into the gynecology unit looking for a woman they "wanted," going curtain to curtain on a thirty-bed ward until the cops came to chase them away. At Jacobi, an Italian gentleman I was treating after his heart attack had a special room at the end of the hall through which a parade of people passed, some of them kneeling to kiss his ring. When he left the hospital, he took me aside, gave me a box of De Nobili cigars, and told me I'd never have to lock the door to my apartment again.

I should say something about the rest of the world, but the truth was, I barely had time to notice. Back in medical school, during the first two basic-science years, I'd go back to our little apartment within walking distance of the hospital and sit on the couch with my wife, home from her day at Columbia University. It was 1973. Together we watched the Watergate hearings and caught all the dramatic moments—"There is a cancer on the presidency!"—and most days, we also caught the travails of the soap opera characters of *Somerset.* But now my soap operas, such as they were, could be seen live on the wards: the adulterous nurse and resident having sex in the on-call room, the resident stealing prescription drugs from the nurses' station, the stab victim dropped at the door of the ER.

It was with some sadness that I left the Bronx for New Haven, where life would be more cerebral but less dramatic (and less playful). Still, I was ready for subspecialty training. My wife noticed that my house-staff years had taken a toll: when I wasn't on call, I was asleep. She was okay about it because she was getting her PhD in English literature and was pretty busy herself. She said we should wait to have kids until she had her degree, only it wasn't just about the degree; it was because I was so absent during those years. But I didn't consider my exhaustion unusual. Wasn't everybody taking to their beds the moment they came home?

Those blood sugars were nothing. A blip. I wasn't sick. Not me.

Mrs. Delancey, with gap teeth and ebony skin, wearing a flowered dress and a black patch over one eye, says she's just fine "except for the high blood and the sugar diabetes." Fine, that is, except not fine: high blood pressure, high glucose, plus advanced kidney disease. She also has had mucormycosis, a fungus that affects diabetics who have ketoacidosis, particularly their eyes and nasal passages. The fungus has eaten out half her face.

I say, for the umpteenth time, that dialysis will help correct the symptoms of kidney failure and restore her appetite.

"You know how I feel," she says.

The facts haven't made much of an impression on her; the fact, for example, that renal failure is likely to kill her. She's a lovely person: warm, kind, devout. Maybe it's her spiritual beliefs that have made her reject treatment? Whatever it is, she is adamant: no dialysis.

"Would it be all right for me to go to Mississippi?" she asks. "I got family down there."

She means, go home to die. I say, "Of course."

It was during my fellowship in kidney medicine at Yale that I began to understand that "cure" was an elusive concept. One of the things that had attracted me to nephrology was the fact that sometimes you could actually make someone better. Toward the end of my residency in internal medicine, when I was deciding which sub-specialty to enter, I almost chose neurology—I loved the intricate science of the brain—but I found it depressing clinically. Identify the brain lesion, and then what? There wasn't much you could do about a stroke, a brain tumor, a closed head injury; at least not in the seventies. But the kidney was control central, critical for maintaining the body's physiological balance. With the kidney, you got the feeling you could fix things; all you had to do was identify the imbalance and correct it.

It was Fred Finkelstein, my first attending physician at Yale, who introduced me to the wonders of renal physiology. Early on in my fellowship, he showed me a patient suffering from dehydration, and I'd never seen such a low urine sodium—that is, he was retaining salt rather than dumping it in the urine. The salt retention caused the body to retain water, too, thereby preventing further dehydration. It was amazing to me that the body could maintain its homeostasis so cleverly. How did it do that? Fred told me, in a tone of awe, "It's the collecting duct." I felt in awe myself: *the collecting duct.*

I was extremely interested in the "ins" and "outs" of maintaining the body's equilibrium, and the kidney is responsible for much of this. Its key job is to shuttle ions like sodium, potassium, calcium, chloride, and bicarbonate back and forth across highly specialized membranes, reabsorbing some electrolytes back into the body, excreting others in the urine. Exquisitely responsive to imbalances, the kidney is constantly correcting, or attempting to correct, concentrations that are too high or too low. And sometimes, you, the nephrologist, could step in where the kidney was failing, correct the electrolytes, and (cue the trumpets!) cure the patient.

Still, despite the electrolyte wizardry, and despite the wonders of modern drugs and modern technology, nephrology wasn't all magnificent reasoning and miracle cures. Our box of fix-its was imperfect. Take dialysis, a mechanical means of cleansing the blood of waste products, which a certain number of patients in kidney failure—uremic, suffering from accumulated toxins, cognitively impaired—would refuse despite the prospect of imminent death. Even on dialysis, there were some patients who couldn't stand life hooked to "the machine." Another problem was kidney transplantation, not a panacea, even if it looked like one. Early on in my fellowship, I saw a teenage kid who'd had a transplant that cured him of his renal disease. He was being treated with corticosteroids to suppress his immune system and prevent his body from rejecting the organ, plus minoxidil for hypertension. When his body grew massive and he sprouted hair all over, his friends started to call him the Incredible Hulk. He got depressed, stopped his meds, and lost the kidney that had been donated to him.

Death was always there, lurking around the next corner, even in a nephrology fellowship, where we were mostly dialyzing people, correcting electrolytes, prescribing drugs. But despite the ongoing threat of a life-or-death crisis, it was during my fellowship that I slowly, patient by patient, began to grasp the meaning of what it means to be chronically ill. At Jacobi, I'd taken care of acutely sick city hospital patients, treating major multisystem disease in a generally older population. House-staff interventions were critical to the immediate survival of people who had no private physicians. I loved the sense of responsibility and power: I was the one who could make all the difference. What I didn't have much sense of was the ongoing lives of the patients after discharge, except on the rare occasions when I got involved in the social medicine side of things, insuring that the patient's apartment had heat or making a home visit to check on medications. I have to confess, I liked the crisis environment; the sense of turning a situation around and actively fixing something.

But a big difference at Yale was that I began to see the patients as larger than the sum of their admissions. What had happened to them before they got to me? What might happen to them after they left me? These questions began to register more strongly. Looking at lab values and ruminating about physiological processes, I would think, "Hey, just fix it." But things weren't always as fixable as I'd hoped.

I found out that sometimes it's no-win, no matter what you do. I came up against the hard decisions required to sustain a life over the long haul—the weighing and balancing that can help someone re- cover from setbacks, accept the unimaginable; even, sometimes, ac- cept the end of trying. Over time, case by case, I've built something like a personal philosophy. Young doctors take the Hippocratic oath, which famously says *Primum non nocere*: "First do no harm." It's a good beginning, but it doesn't really say it all. Doing nothing can be harmful. Sometimes, to do good, you have to get in there, risk side effects and consequences, push for active treatment. At the same time, pushing treatment can, depending on the circumstances, cause harm: prolong suffering, exact too high a price, gratify the doctor more than the patient. Untangling these knots can take a lifetime.

With kidney disease, I was beginning to see that the art is often in helping someone live with it, not in curing it.

Carl Baldwin is a mild-mannered man: white shirt, bow tie, creased pants, combed hair. Although he has been diagnosed with chronic undifferentiated schizophrenia, he shows no signs of mental illness. He has another disease, too: diabetes insipidus, caused by the lithium he takes to treat his mental illness. He was one of the first to get lithium back in the 1960s. Now, twenty years later, he produces over fifteen liters of urine per day, and needs to drink that much just to replace his fluid losses.

I ask him how the urination affects him.

Mr. Baldwin looks distressed. "I can't take a bus across town—I have to get out along the way two or three times. I've learned where all the bathrooms and water fountains are on the route. It's embarrassing at work; I have to go to the bathroom every half hour." He shifts in his chair, jiggles his foot. "I've tried putting a catheter on my penis to collect my urine—I tie a bag to my leg."

Poor Mr. Baldwin. Every half hour, all day long, all night long, day in, day out. How can he think? How can he live?

"That sounds pretty terrible." I lean forward. "Would you consider coming off of lithium?"

He immediately says, "No."

"Can you say why not?"

"I can't risk it. Nothing could ever be as bad as the hospitalizations."

Whatever his mind had been like two decades ago, he wasn't going back there, ever.

Carl Baldwin's feelings were understandable. Before going on lithium, he'd come into the hospital numerous times, psychotic and disoriented, but once on the drug, he became productive and worked full time, without a single hospitalization in two decades. Nephrologists see lots of people on lithium, because one of its complications is kidney disease, including this type of diabetes, in-sipidus, a condition that causes resistance to antidiuretic hormone

(ADH), creating massive thirst and voluminous urination. Diabetes insipidus (DI) is an entirely different disease from diabetes mellitus (DM). *Insipidus* means "bland"; *mellitus,* "sweet" (or "honeyed"). The names are a tip-off that, once upon a time, these diagnoses were made by taste. (One elderly patient with diabetes mellitus was "diagnosed" by his wife, who found a trail of ants walking on the floor to the toilet bowl—flies to the honey pot.) The word *diabetes,* from the Greek for "passing through," indicates that the one (and only) thing diabetes insipidus and diabetes mellitus have in common is excessive discharge of urine.

Carl Baldwin wasn't going to trade diabetes insipidus for the chaos of psychosis. The mind and body are a continuum, and sometimes you pay a price here to get a benefit there. I told him we'd get together with his psychiatrist to talk over his treatment and how we could help him manage.

I often think of Mr. Baldwin with his urine bag tied to his leg, holding on to his sanity with both hands. When I see patients with schizophrenia or manic depression on lithium, I never say, "We have to take you off the drug." But I don't underestimate what it costs them to stay on it. Once I saw a schizophrenic patient who had been put in restraints because of his huge liquid intake. He had a chair on his back as he tried to stagger toward the sink for a drink.

Other medical conditions also put people between a rock and a hard place. Sometimes, there just isn't a good solution.

———

Maya Lichinsky sits across from me, a hat shading half her face. Pink wormlike scars nest in the half of her face that's visible. She's been taking immunosuppressive drugs to prevent rejection of her kidney transplant, but the price has been high: a series of disfiguring oral surgeries for the cancers that have developed on the drug regimen. Now the cancer has recurred in her mouth.

"The surgeons tell me they might have to remove my tongue." Her face is in shadow. Is she crying? She sounds remarkably calm.

I lean toward her, upset. "If we take you off the drugs, maybe the cancer won't spread." I don't say it, but we both know that stopping the immunosuppression means she'll lose the kidney.

"I won't do it," she says. Her words are faintly slurred.

Well, of course not, I think; no surgery. Who could accept the loss of speech? But I'm thinking wrong. It's dialysis she's saying no to—the dialysis that is her fate once the transplant has failed. Not only does she hate dialysis, but she values her transplanted kidney, a gift from her sister. Sacrificing the kidney and returning to dialysis are definitely out. For the woman sitting across from me, surgery—more scars, half a tongue, no tongue—is okay by comparison.

"I'll take my chances with cancer," she says.

In the course of my career, I've struggled with many situations like this and have concluded that my role is to accept the patient's choice. When I think it's a wrong decision, I weigh in with my opinion, but I'm not an enforcer. In the end, after the discussions, the encouragement, the posing of possibilities, you have to respect a person's wishes. You can't insist on dialysis, you can't insist on taking away the toxic drug that also helps, you can't tell someone to give up her transplant. At the same time, I'm not a big fan of sitting by while a patient tells me that he's abandoning the fight. I really do feel optimistic that things can be better; that by pulling together, a patient and I can make it more bearable. Do-not-resuscitate orders tend to bother me. I sometimes think patients feel badgered when you ask them about DNR, as though you're subtly encouraging them to just die already. At the same time, I know that people need to give directions about how they want to be treated.

I remember an intern who was taking care of a man with schizophrenia in renal failure. The intern reported that when he asked the man if he wanted to choose dialysis or accept death from uremia, the man decided to be dialyzed—but, the intern explained to me, the man might not be competent to make that decision. Personally, I don't think it works in that direction.

And what about coma? How do you decide, and who decides, whether it's the end of the road? Occasionally, surprising recoveries do happen. There's a joke about a man who falls into a coma in 1958 and wakes up in 1972. He asks the medical student how President Eisenhower is doing, and the student replies, "I'm sorry to say that President Eisenhower is dead."

"Oh, no!" the man says. "That means Nixon is president!"

So what is my philosophy? Do I believe in extreme measures? Do I believe in stopping treatment when quality of life is diminished? The answer is, it depends. I try to help patients live if it's the right thing for them, and I try to help them face death if it's not. Patients are asking what I think, but they're also telling me what they think. I'm willing to listen.

After a year as a clinical fellow, I moved into the laboratory in order to study renal transport: processes of reabsorption and secretion. The lab was a relief after the pressures of clinical medicine. If you came in late, the worst that could happen was that the experiment would occur somewhat later in the day. After a seven-year sprint, I finally had some time with my wife. We had one son, and then, two years later, on the eve of our departing for Harvard Medical School, a second one. I felt as though life were opening up in front of me; as though I were just beginning.

We're climbing Sleeping Giant Mountain—not really much of a mountain, but hulking enough to earn its name. We have the baby in the backpack and Andrew is in the stroller, which is pretty useless on the steep paths and twisting trails. My wife and I trade off holding his hand, carrying him. We come out of a patch of trees into a small meadow strewn with boulders; the sun is blazing. Suddenly I'm light-headed, dizzy. I sit down on a flat rock, my pulse racing, my vision fading in and out. I can hear the baby crying. My wife's already handing me Life Savers, and I eat one after the other, panicked. We sit there awhile. Andrew is getting restless. "Come on, Daddy, let's go!"

Now I'm feeling hot, irritable, itchy. What's all this about? Low blood sugar, and then an overshoot?

Maybe it's just exertion. Maybe it's just nerves.

2

My Name Is Lucy Rooney

Lucy Rooney, a young woman with dark hair, blue eyes, and red cheeks, sits across the desk from me—the picture of health, but not healthy. She has a bad, potentially fatal, disease. I'd had an angiogram done, looking for fibromuscular dysplasia, which classically presents in a woman her age as new-onset severe hypertension with low potassium. But what I found was something worse. Lucy has PAN—polyarteritis nodosa—an inflammatory process that affects many vessels in the body, particularly the larger blood vessels, or arteries. PAN also causes nodes (nodosa) to form in the branches of the circulatory system. Lucy is plenty sick—she came into the hospital with a skyrocketing blood pressure that could have killed her on the spot—but she's eager for all the details, including the medical nomenclature. She seems highly organized, very intelligent. She doesn't look scared, sitting there across from me. In fact, she's just been telling me how lucky she feels that the elevated blood pressure was picked up on a routine gynecological exam; that she hasn't died of a heart attack or a stroke.

When I've explained what her angiogram shows, Lucy wants to take a look at what she calls her "funky little aneurysms." After we've looked at the images, we sit down again.

Lucy gives me a smile. "So, Doc, how long do I have to live?"

"We're going to treat you with Cytoxan."

"Come again?"

"A chemotherapy drug."

"I have cancer?"

"Chemotherapy isn't just for cancer. It helps reduce the systemic inflammation."

"And then, ta-dah, my hair falls out. Anything else?"

I don't like having to tell her this last part. "Well, you could lose your ovarian function."

Her face loses the smile. "Why is that?"

"Your ovaries are releasing eggs every month, and the Cytoxan likes to go where the action is."

Lucy leans forward. "This is really important, Dr. S. Really important. I want to have kids if I survive this."

I tell her that along with the chemo, we'll try Lupron, a new drug that reduces blood flow to the ovaries and also acts as an antagonist to gonadotrophins, turning off hormonal activity and creating a temporary menopause. This "time-out" may protect the ovaries from the effects of the chemo and preserve reproductive function later on.

"Okay, then." She adjusts herself in the chair, reaches across the desk to shake my hand. "We have a deal."

Lucy was one of my patients at Brigham and Women's Hospital in Boston, where I ran nephrology clinics and taught students and house staff as a young instructor and researcher at Harvard Medical School. A lot happened before this office visit, and a lot came after. Some of it I was there for, some Lucy told me about, and some she wrote about in a personal case report. I'm going to piece together Lucy's story for you, using her own words as much as possible, because her experience reveals so much about the struggle to hold on to identity when mind and body are under assault from illness.

To set the record straight, Lucy isn't her real name; it's Sheila. Sheila invented Lucy Rooney at a low point in her illness, and since then, Lucy has become Sheila's stand-in—a character in her own right. Lucy is an interesting and useful invention: a symbol of the selfhood that Sheila preserved, and in a sense discovered, during the course of her battle with PAN.

Sheila's story begins with a visit to her gynecologist for a routine checkup. The first hint of trouble was when the nurse's eyes bulged out as she read the blood pressure cuff. A second assistant came in—ditto—and finally the gynecologist, who sent her straight to the emergency room. Sheila hadn't even felt ill, except for some headaches she treated with over-the-counter ibuprofen. At age thirty-one, she was full steam ahead, no worries. Even now she didn't feel worried. It was all too surreal. She "tootled" downstairs to the ER, where they put nifedipine capsules under her tongue to bring down the pressure; she was nauseous and vomiting. When, around midnight, the intern suggested that maybe she could go home and come back in the morning, Sheila told him she'd wrap her car around a tree on Memorial Drive if he let her drive. That was the moment it dawned on her that she was really sick.

As the renal attending that month, I met Sheila the next morning, with a team that included a rheumatologist, two fellows, a resident, and an intern. Sheila was good-natured, funny. "Whatever," she said. "I'm sure you guys can fix it." We did the workup, including the angiogram showing the "funky aneurysms," and then tried to get her pressure down with antihypertensives. But after a two-week hospitalization during which the blood pressure didn't budge, the team put her on a six-month schedule of monthly infusions of Cytoxan.

The Cytoxan was a wake-up call, Sheila says; at last she realized that she had a big-time diagnosis, a wild-sounding disease. These were wild days altogether. Her hospitalization was the longest break she'd taken from work in four years. (She ran her own translation service, In Other Words.) Would she be able to keep working if she remained so ill? And, in what would become a very important subplot of her story, what would happen to her ovaries? Would they be "ovaries flambés"?

Even so, Sheila says she felt lucky. When she went to the infusion suite, a lot of the other patients had cancer and were on much bigger doses of chemo than she was taking. She didn't experience any nausea at first, and when she suffered some severe bouts after a few months on Cytoxan, the antinausea drug Zofran mitigated the bad side effect. The nurses were great, and she had the perk of flying high on the corticosteroid drug prednisone to offset the downer of the chemo. Of course, sometimes she didn't know who she was exactly—or, as she puts it, "which Sheila was going to show up." She felt similarly about the Lupron. Because of its influence on hormones, the drug spun her around: her mood was up, down, and sideways. When she finally got off the Cytoxan and the prednisone, she felt like, "Oh, look, I'm back."

Sheila did feel that her life had turned upside down in the course of what became three years of treatment; she says she had to recognize at a pretty young age that there are things you have no control over. She spent some time looking for the underlying cause of her illness, but with PAN, as with a lot of diseases, "you don't get an answer." The search for a cause was really, she says, a search for some form of control, and she spent a number of years obsessively recording her blood pressure—the one sign that could help her doctors track what was going on with her.

She regarded certain things that happened along the way as mere bumps in the road. At one point, HPV, human papillomavirus, emerged in a particularly aggressive form because she was immunosuppressed; the lesions had to be surgically excised in an operating room instead of via office laser because the virus was in the vaginal wall and on the cervix. When she got the news, Sheila didn't even cry. She joked with the scheduling nurse, "Just put it on the list."

And then there was her long-running concern with saving her reproductive capacity. After six months of Cytoxan, the radiologist said, "Everything looks clean," at which point Sheila posted a note on my office door: "I have kidneys of bronze, but hopefully I have ovaries of steel. See, I'm not even sick! Ha ha!" It was then the team sat her down, all of us wearing what she describes as "poker faces," to break the bad news: she needed another two years of Cytoxan, at quarterly intervals, to ensure the remission. Sheila says it hit her like a ton of bricks. When she said, "Hey, look at my scans, I'm doing well," we had to tell her that years ago, when there was no Cytoxan to offer, people usually died of PAN. "Okay, guys, that's good, that's enough," she said. "I don't need to hear any more."

It was then that she turned her full attention to reproduction: a distraction from her anxiety about PAN, and a drama all its own.

She had a serious boyfriend, and she'd just begun to think, Maybe I do want to have kids. The boyfriend stuck around for nine months of PAN and, *bam,* he was outta there. Until then, they'd been seeing a fertility specialist who recommended creating an embryo. The science wasn't in place to freeze eggs, because without the chorion (the membrane surrounding an embryo), the egg couldn't survive. But they could freeze an embryo using her boyfriend's sperm. It would be an insurance policy in case her ovaries failed in the longer run. But the boyfriend was dragging his feet; he didn't show up for appointments with the social worker, he wouldn't go for sperm analysis. Finally, Sheila said to him, "Are you in the boat or out of the boat? Are you holding an oar? Are you paddling in the same direction as me?" The boyfriend said he'd heard from a doctor pal of his that people who go through Cytoxan had an 80 percent survival rate—so his question to her was, did she have seventy-nine friends or nineteen friends?

Sheila says this was the low point for her: thirty-three years old, her ovaries going up in smoke, and not a man in sight. Add to that, her fertility specialist was completely tone-deaf. He kept saying, "Gamete preservation is the way to go," and pushing the idea of donor sperm, when sperm donation was not something that Sheila would consider. She wasn't the typical career woman with an agenda: "and now it's time for a baby, check." She wanted a baby only if she was creating life within a family. The person she had kids with—if she ever could have kids—would have to be really special. What if she died? He would have to be a great dad. Even if she was just a permanently sick person, maybe it wouldn't be fair to the child if she wouldn't be able to mother it.

As for the frozen embryo, if she had this piece of tissue in a freezer somewhere, she would feel responsible for it. When, or if, she found her life partner and then, quite possibly, couldn't conceive on her own, she'd be asking him to raise a child who wasn't his.

While she was doing all this self-questioning, the fertility guy acknowledged to her that he'd never actually implanted a frozen embryo that had led to a successful pregnancy. Basically she thought he was saying, be a guinea pig.

There was a certain amount of guinea pig in everything that happened to Sheila: the Cytoxan was a fairly new protocol, the Lupron was "off-label" (employed for a use not yet approved by the U.S. Food and Drug Administration), the Zofran for nausea was new, the frozen embryo option was new. Mostly she didn't mind. Cytoxan? Sure. Lupron? You bet. But she wasn't going to mess with inseminating and then banking eggs for a spot in the freezer section. She says she felt the words *Imperfect* and *Unworthy* were written on her forehead.

A few things helped her at this point. First, she consulted a reproductive specialist who told her the dose of Cytoxan wasn't large enough to wipe out her ovaries. Second, she allowed herself to hope that the Lupron would do what it was advertised to do and protect her fertility. I asked her if she wanted to see a psychologist—I was really worried about her depression—but she said she was too busy to pee, much less talk with someone. Sheila wasn't telling her clients that she was ill, and she kept meeting deadlines while working around the chemo.

But the "no therapy" led to an interesting development. During this same rough stretch, she left a note on my door, trying not to bother me during an office visit; it turned into what she calls a "long-tailed note" that "tipped you to a lot more in me than would have come up in a clinic appointment." It was a genuine, moving account: I got to hear about how crushed she felt by the deadbeat boyfriend and the tone-deaf fertility specialist, and I also heard, in her words, what it felt like to fall suddenly sick and go through three years of exhausting tests, treatments, reevaluations, all with a brooding sense of urgency and uncertainty. The note stuck in my mind, and I asked if she'd like to write up something for the medical students. At Harvard, we were creating a curriculum called the New Pathway, a tutorial approach to disease that used actual cases in order to prepare first- and second-year students for the clinical experiences up ahead.

Sheila said something like "Wow, yeah." And that's when, as she puts it, "Lucy Rooney reared her head." Expanding on her "long-tailed note," she "oozed out" forty pages of prose that expressed all her hurt and anger, as well as the facts of her illness. Together we tried to figure out how to turn those pages into something teachable, and came up with the idea of alternating her experience as a patient with chart notes written by The Doctor. It was Sheila who suggested one font for her personal account and another for the notes in the chart. As a translator and linguist, she was very alert to the "two tongues."

Here's a brief excerpt from "My Name Is Lucy Rooney," the New Pathway teaching case:

My name is Lucy Rooney, I'm 31 years old, and I've always thought of myself as a hale-and-hearty type. When I went for my gynecological checkup, just the touring bit with Pap-smear-and-breast-exam-to-go, it turned out I was at least a space shuttle ride from good health. All I'd had to tip me off were some bad headaches that would wake me up at 4:00 a.m. if I hadn't taken my usual three ibuprofen at 11:00 p.m. But you could see the gynecologist's jaw drop when she took my blood pressure—she looked as though she thought the cuff was broken. Come to find out the blood pressure was 210/140 and the headaches were only a symptom of a more serious disease process at work. I was admitted to College Hospital that day, and since a diagnosis was made, my life hasn't been the same.

And here's The Doctor talking:

This was the first CH admission for a 31-year-old white female linguist with frontal headaches, nausea of two weeks' duration, and severe hypertension noted by her gynecologist. She denies fatigue, fever, blurred vision, abdominal pain, and myalgias. Her blood pressure four months before admission was 130/80 and all previous BPs were normal. Two years ago, she was seen by her physician for arthralgias in her ankles, but there is no other history of arthritis. Over the past eighteen months, she has had a recurrent reticular rash of the lower extremities. Medications include birth control pills and tetracycline for acne. There is no family history of hypertension.

Physical examination revealed a well-appearing young woman, blood pressure 210/140 mm Hg in both arms, fundoscopic exam was normal, lungs were clear, cardiac exam revealed II/VI systolic ejection murmur, abdomen was nontender without hepatosplenomegaly, stool was guaiac negative, neurologic and musculoskeletal exams were normal. Lower extremities revealed livedo reticularis.

Labs: K 3.5 HCO3 29 BUN 15 Cr 0.9 hematocrit 39 WBC 10,100 U/A 1+ protein and benign sediment erythrocyte sed rate 56 mm/hr.

It's obvious even from this short excerpt that doctors are trained to talk to other doctors. According to legend, upon graduating from medical school, a doctor will have acquired a vocabulary of nearly fifty-five thousand new words.[3] It requires a concerted effort to translate all that jargon back into words that intersect with the patient's actual experience of body and self.

Lucy tells what her actual experience felt like. She writes about her discomfort with the angiogram, which takes "just about forever"; meanwhile, the radiology resident, though apparently fascinated by her kidneys, is oblivious to the real her on the table. She draws some solace from the fact that she's an interesting case, with the requisite "three heads" to merit the attention of a whole parade of specialists. When she finally hears her diagnosis, PAN, she thinks it sounds "like a brand of peanut butter or a mythological allusion." She worries about "pan-fried ovaries" and the "Big Long-Term Issues, of being totally dominated by the disease 'thing,' feeling dependent on doctors, wondering if I'll have a shortened life expectancy—and just feeling sick of feeling sick." And she states her working philosophy: "one day at a time, carpe diem, life-is-uncertain-eat-dessert-first. So far so good."

Lucy/Sheila is one of a number of patients who have taught the medical students a way of looking at disease that includes, centrally, the person who has it. The tutor guide to the case helped the medical students identify the traits that enabled her to deal successfully with a catastrophic illness. She's funny, for one thing, and for another, she's got a lot of grit. The days of being hale and hearty may be over, but she's not down and out. She's a fighter. Submitting to a tough chemotherapy regimen, she manages to hang on to a sense of herself. She knows she's interesting to all these intrusive doctors, and she has her own opinions about them—the radiology resident may be an uncaring jerk, but she likes some of us. She also benefits from telling her story to the students (as they too benefit from hearing it). She's the one this is happening to: Lucy Rooney, a person with a name.

About six years after her final dose of Cytoxan, Sheila was the final exam for the second-year pathophysiology course, one hundred eighty medical students in a lecture hall asking her questions, including "What's your diagnosis?" In the interim, she married an old college friend. (Seventeen years after they met, it seemed like a good idea to kiss; then it seemed like a *really* good idea.) And then, miracle, she conceived her daughter. She was eight months pregnant at the time of the final exam, representing a case of "sudden-onset hypertension in a young woman." She says she feels she was a "good visual."

Sheila invented Lucy to tell her story, and the act of "telling" turned out to be a way of putting together all that had happened to her. Through Lucy, Sheila could portray the self that she'd become in the course of her battle. Most critically, "Lucy Rooney" was able to sustain a sense of personal agency and worth in the face of chronic illness. Implicit in Lucy's story is how tempting it is to give in to the diagnosis, to let yourself be reduced to the thing you have. Lucy made it her business to pay minimal attention to her PAN diagnosis, preferring instead to record blood pressures, keep up with her translating business, and fight for her ovaries. But "becoming your disease" is encouraged by the medical environment: you walk into a hospital, and they take away your clothes, hand you a cotton gown, slap on a plastic bracelet with an ID number. Doctors talking to each other in elevators will refer to the "heart failure" in room 12, the "appendicitis" on floor 6, the "malignant melanoma" on the oncology unit. With HIPAA—the Health Insurance Portability and Accountability Act of 1996, which established new privacy regulations protecting patients from the careless broadcasting of personal information by health professionals—such shorthand has become necessary. But even if privacy is the newer justification, I think that doctors, for their own reasons—because they're jaded or busy— often use such references to distance themselves and turn a person into a "case." Sometimes you see language in charts like "Thanks for the interesting consult," or "This fascinating case of . . ." I've never felt comfortable saying that someone's personal tragedy is a "great case."

If there's a lesson here, and of course there is, it's this: you are not your illness. You have an individual story to tell. You have a name, a history, a personality. Staying yourself is part of the battle.[4]

Lucy's story has a happy ending. Sheila says at some point in the last eight years she crossed the border into the land of the well. She no longer records blood pressures, and she no longer expects the other shoe to drop every time she comes for her annual checkup. She even serves as a community member on the Human Research Committee that I chair; the HRC evaluates clinical trials at the hospital according to ethical guidelines, and considers such things as informed consent and patient risk. Sheila's many experiences with experimental treatments have made her an especially good contributor.

Given her prognosis, Sheila is a rare success story. But it's not the end of the story that's the only important thing here. It's how Sheila lived with her disease, how she developed a narrative of herself (or of "Lucy") in the course of many shocks and threats, and how she communicated all this to me and to the medical students. In the course of my long career, I've seen many people battle their illnesses, and I've come to see that each person writes a narrative as individual as a thumbprint. Some stories are about successful adaptation or, happiest of all, about conquering the foe; others are darker, more tangled, more troubled. But every story deserves respect. Every story has a real, actual teller, and needs to be listened to.

As for me, I can't say that in my early years I did as well as Lucy Rooney. I didn't want the story I was in.

~

The patient is young, just starting out his medical career. He looks pale, exhausted, drawn. He says he's been losing weight; also, he's thirsty all the time, urinating a lot. Sometimes he gets waves of dizziness, like he's going to pass out, and other times he feels sluggish, like he can barely stay awake. He's thinking that whatever it is might be related to the stress of his first academic job. Or maybe it's a pheochromocytoma.

Pheo? He's got to be kidding. What he's described doesn't sound like an adrenaline-producing tumor. Poor guy. "If you were sitting on my side of the desk, what would you think?"

The young man looks unhappy. "A horse, not a zebra."

The finger stick shows a blood glucose of 400. "You need insulin."

"How about an oral hypoglycemic?"

"You're very symptomatic. The only thing that's going to help is injections."

"Can my wife give the shots?"

"What is she, a nurse?"

"No, she teaches."

"You're going to have to learn to do this yourself. After a while, it's like brushing your teeth."

The young man ponders this for a moment. How independent does he have to be, facing this illness? How alone is he in his own body?

He leaves the office in a hurry. Doctors make the worst patients.

~

That was no patient. That was me. I'd had an upper respiratory illness at the end of the summer, right before I started a research career at Harvard Medical School, and though the cold cleared up, I felt sicker and sicker. One evening in the fall, I was lying on the living room couch of our rented house—the baby asleep, Andrew playing in his bedroom—listening to the sounds of my wife making dinner. When she came to get me, I told her I was dying.

I couldn't think clearly. Excessive thirst and urination, weight loss, cognitive confusion: this was not rocket science. Most likely it was the high blood sugar clouding my brain, but I still wasn't buying. Maybe this was all a mistake. Maybe it was some other disease. Maybe I could take a pill. Maybe my wife could give the injections. I was way too busy for this.

And I certainly wasn't going to be testing my blood sugars very often. Glucometers were fairly new back then, big clunky things with thick lancets that hurt like hell. Urine dipsticks were the more usual method of testing, and they were notoriously unreliable. No, I couldn't be bothered with all that.[5]

I made one accommodation: I injected insulin once a day. And that was it for a very long time.

Coming to Harvard—my first real job, doing research in the renal division, seeing patients at Brigham and Women's Hospital, teaching at Harvard Medical School—meant I'd arrived professionally. But it turned out to be more of a struggle than I'd imagined. The lab was demanding: suddenly I was running a whole operation, overseeing the experiments of fellows, doing paperwork, handling money, counting glassware, ordering animals. I was better at the science than the housekeeping. Eventually I switched tracks, focusing on clinical trials rather than laboratory research, and spending more time with students and patients.

Lucy Rooney was one of the early patients I saw, and the way she told her story proved very illuminating not only to the medical students but to me. There were others, too, dating from that period, who told the stories of their illness in distinctive, constructive ways.

Tom Mahon clasps his hands on his round belly and leans toward me. "So, Doc, let's talk about what I've got. This ADPKD thing." Tom has recently been hospitalized for renal colic—acute pain, urine the color of cranberry juice—and an ultrasound showed a renal cyst measuring fourteen centimeters in diameter. That's five and a half inches.

"You know what the letters stand for?"

"Something, something, something, kidney disease."

"Autosomal dominant polycystic kidney disease." *I'm reminded of a* New Yorker *cartoon: the doctor sitting opposite the patient and informing him, "You have a condition whose name is very hard to remember."*

"Right," *Tom says.* "Tell me about that."

"Let's back up for a minute. Does anyone else in the family have health problems?"

"I'm an amateur genealogist; I've filled in the whole family tree. I should know what everyone died of, but I never thought about it. Let's see. My mother, she died of a stroke. My uncle died of kidney failure. My cousin had an early heart attack. There was an aunt who had something too, I can't remember what." *He seems surprised by his own list.* "They were dropping like flies for a while there. Then there's my brothers. They're going strong, I think—we don't communicate much—but they have some sort of kidney trouble."

"That's the ADPKD," *I tell him.*

Tom looks shocked. "But it was really just Uncle George. The doctors never said what he had, exactly, but I remember my mother made me watch him when he napped. He used to nod off and drop his cigarette on the carpet. I liked him, but he smelled like urine."

"It's likely all these deaths are connected." I explain to Tom that his family carries a genetic mutation that changes the composition of the kidney, causing cysts to form, raising blood pressure, creating brain aneurysms. Often the disease doesn't show up until a person is in his thirties; it takes decades for the genetic defect to manifest in enlarged cysts. Not everyone in the family would have the defect, but he clearly does, and his two brothers too, probably.

"So, Doc, what's going to happen to me?"

"Things are a lot better now than they used to be. In the U.S., almost no one dies of uremia anymore. We have dialysis now, for one thing."

Tom looks scared.

"And a whole other bag of tricks," I add quickly.

Dialysis is the specter that haunts everyone who has kidney disease, but whatever its drawbacks, the first thing to recognize is what a lifesaver it was when it first appeared on the scene in the 1940s. But it wasn't until the 1960s that dialysis became clinically practical for large numbers of people in the States. It was then that an outpatient unit with six dialysis machines opened at the University of Washington Hospital in Seattle. It was a dramatic moment: you'd live if you had access to the machine, you'd die without it. In the early days, when sick people were lining up for the very few machines available, two patients arrived at the renal clinic in a Bronx hospital. A committee had been set up to make the difficult decisions about who would get access to the single machine available. The two men in kidney failure both had wives and children; however, only one of them had life insurance. The committee's decision was to dialyze the man without life insurance. These sorts of wrenching decisions are no longer necessary, now that dialysis is available to anyone who needs it. (A federal End Stage Renal Disease program, established in 1972, makes dialysis a public entitlement covered by Medicare and ensures that a significant proportion of health care funding goes to the creation and maintenance of dialysis units.)

Tom grew up in a different era, and saw family members die prematurely from polycystic disease. Uncle George, falling asleep in his chair, dropping lit cigarettes, smelling of accumulated toxins, hadn't lived long enough to benefit from the advent of dialysis. For Tom, though, dialysis was a terrifying prospect. A physician's assistant had shown him and his wife Anna around the Brigham unit at some point after his diagnosis—"Just looking," he joked with the nurses—and they were both frightened of the sci-fi look of the machine with its convoluted tubes and vials, and of the patients with fistulas in their arms—scarred places where a vein and artery had been joined together for ready IV access. There was something eerie about the whole thing, Tom said, all those people lying around hooked to machines, dependent on the damn things just to stay alive.

In medical parlance, dialysis is referred to as the "black box": the magic machine that sustains life after kidneys have failed. The tools of my trade, office nephrology, aren't as fancy, but they are magical another way. With medications, supplements, lifestyle adjustments, it's possible to keep kidneys going, and to keep people off dialysis, for a long time; sometimes forever.

Tom, it seems, isn't likely to need dialysis soon. Not only does he take his meds religiously, keep all his office appointments, and submit to regular ultrasounds and other tests, but he's also made himself an expert on ADPKD. He reads journal articles and follows the research on experimental drugs that may inhibit cyst formation. Tom also knows all about his creatinine, potassium, and blood urea nitrogen (BUN)—the chief measures of his kidney function. Beyond that, he's expanded his study of his family's genealogy all the way back to Ireland in 1806, marking in the spaces of relatives who likely died from the ravages of polycystic disease, which include stroke and heart attack as well as kidney failure. Tom is a contractor, who likes to fix things. No-salt diet? No problem. Antihypertensives? Okay. Watch the red meat? You got it. Compliance hasn't been an issue for Tom.

He seems to have avoided the swinging axe that lopped off so many branches of his family tree. His eagerness to understand and control his illness has made him a great collaborator in his own treatment. Together we've worked hard to manage the ups and downs of kidneys that don't function normally. At my request, he's put together a lecture for the medical students, including genealogic illustrations, which he's presented often over the years. Most recently, he's shared his experiences and expertise with a PhD student studying the genetic mutations involved in polycystic disease.[6]

Like Lucy Rooney, Tom has found a way to tell his own story, in his own voice. He's a funny, personable guy who makes friends easily and gets along with hospital staff. He has a mildly satiric view of some of the medical receptionists, who tend to be young and callous, but he says at least they've been through "smile training." Though his kidneys have grown in size and developed numerous cysts, he's been remarkably healthy over the last twenty-five years, except for a few kidney stones and one painful episode of gout. The things that bother him most are homely, domestic: the fact that his large kidneys press on his intestines and produce embarrassing stomach rumbles; the fact that, because of the big kidneys, his belly noticeably protrudes. His girth so exceeds his other dimensions that he's been thinking of wearing suspenders to hold his pants up. Anna objects that suspenders will make him seem like an old man, to which Tom replies cheerfully, "I *am* an old man."

Lucy and Tom have both done well with potentially fatal conditions. To what can we attribute their success? The wonders of modern medicine helped: chemotherapy, steroids, medications to control hypertension and cholesterol, corrections of calcium, potassium, and sodium levels. It's also true that Tom has treatment options up ahead that weren't available to the previous generation of his family: not only dialysis and transplant, but a new class of drugs that could alter cyst formation.

So here's to the appropriate application of technology and phar-macology. But there's still something mysterious at work. Other patients with similar diseases and treated according to similar pro-tocols don't respond as well as Lucy and Tom. Is it their "resilience" that makes them survivors? I'm ambivalent about theories of this kind. It's like telling cancer patients to laugh. Sure it's good to laugh, but the flip side is, if you feel depressed—if you fail to "lighten up"—then it's your fault if the disease worsens. This is nonsense.

We rely on science for explanations of what's wrong and how to fix it. Cytoxan for PAN, control of hypertension and diet for ADPKD—what's wrong and how to fix it—are based on an under-standing of vessels, membranes, molecules. But the question "Why me?" haunts everyone who has a bad diagnosis. Beyond the vessels and membranes, there's a deeper cause that's difficult, sometimes impossible, to name. Genetic predisposition provides a bit more of an answer: heredity clearly gave Tom his ADPKD. Even so, some family members escaped the mutation, while others developed a worse form of the disease than Tom's. The preoccupation with lifestyle—what you eat, whether you exercise, do you have bad habits?—is not unlike the search for genetic explanations, only here the cause would be the environment: toxins, foodstuffs, behaviors, substances. But we all know people who smoke, drink, eat Cheez Doodles, lie around on the couch, and live to be one hundred. (I actually had a patient, an Italian shoemaker, who was celebrating his hundredth birthday; when I asked him about his habits, he said he began every day with a breakfast of bacon and eggs.) There's a lot we don't understand, and a lot we can't control. What's in our control can seem almost comical. One study of cholesterol-lowering diets suggests that if you reduced your cholesterol by means of a stringent diet, you'd add three weeks to your life. Too bad the three weeks couldn't be in the middle of your life span, when you could enjoy it. A lot of people (me among them) would conclude, might as well eat lobster.

Our society is notoriously bad at accepting certain painful facts: that we all live in bodies that are subject to time and chance; that health—good or bad—is not fully within our control; that at some point, our bodies will betray us. Barring accidental or violent death, we all die of something. There's another *New Yorker* cartoon, a man contemplating a tombstone that reads, "Never sick a day in his life, and now this." One way or another, the end will come. But as we develop better treatments, the life span increases. More people are living with chronic illness than ever before, with HIV, certain types of cancer, and heart disease becoming, in large measure, chronic conditions.

As Lucy says, in chronic illness, you learn you can't control everything. It's "gonna be what it's gonna be," and all the worry in the world won't change it. But neither Lucy nor Tom used this realistic assessment as the first step on the road to depression or pessimism. They were both willing to try to control what they could. They both hung on to a sense of humor. They were capable of finding pleasure and meaning in life, even while sick. And they developed personal narratives that included, rather than denied, the sick self.

⁓

As a kidney specialist, I see a special subset of the ill: those facing ESRD, or end-stage renal disease. The term, as with so many in medicine, seems designed to terrify people: "end-stage," as though there's nothing afterward. But there is something after kidney function fails, and that something is dialysis. Much of my practice is devoted to staving off the "end" and preventing organ failure. Tom Mahon has been one of the lucky ones, but for many others, dialysis ultimately becomes the only option.

Author James Michener, who was on dialysis for four or five years before he died at the age of ninety, wrote of the adjustments he had to make to conform to what he called the Dialysis Calendar: four-hour sessions occurring on Mondays, Wednesdays, and Fridays, which left him completely exhausted and unable to do life on those days. All business and social activities had to be squeezed into Tuesdays, Thursdays, and weekends. Though Michener expressed his appreciation of dialysis, he longed for the time, not far off, he hoped, when cloned kidneys would replace the intrusive, clumsy, debilitating effects of mechanical intervention. But, on balance, he'd made his peace with what was available to him: "The bottom line of my personal reaction is that even under the rigid dictates of the present system, a reasonably happy life can be achieved if one is willing to meet the system halfway."[7]

But then Michener added a sad story about a "mournful young man," thirty-two years old, who didn't want anything to do with a Dialysis Calendar. The young man chronically reported late for dialysis sessions and left early. Michener reminded him that dialysis was keeping him alive, and that it was possible to live a satisfactory life despite the difficulties. The young man then asked how old he was. Michener replied, "Eighty-seven." The young man gave a scornful laugh; he pointed out that Michener had already lived most of his life and could make the necessary adjustments in his remaining years. But as for himself, he was just starting out, and the thought of living like this terrified him. Shortly thereafter, the young patient stopped coming for dialysis. Shortly after that, he died. Ironically, Michener himself withdrew from dialysis at age 90, when his own quality of life was compromised by mounting medical problems; even so, he lived as well as possible, and for as long as possible, within the strict dictates of the Dialysis Calendar.

It helped that Michener was Michener, and that the burden of dialysis came to him late in life. Meanwhile, the "mournful young man"—a young man without a name, in Michener's telling—felt crushed by the cruel demands placed on him. How do you hang on to your name, yourself, when you live by machines?

John Brice is his usual impeccable self: pin-striped suit and vest, expensive tie and shoes, gold cuff links, and gold watch. He looks like the lawyer he is—polished, professional, except that his skin is pasty, and he's lost some weight. His features are sharp and angled, the suit a little too big in the shoulders. Underneath the aftershave, I catch a whiff of uremia.

Usually straight to the point, his conversation meanders as he de-scribes the last month: he's been falling asleep in the middle of sentences, he forgot two important appointments, his skin feels inflamed, he's having trouble eating. And, oh yes, his younger daughter just graduated from high school. He glimpsed his ex-wife in the audience; the first time he's seen her in two years.

I murmur something about the graduation. There's a pause.

Time to break it to him. "The creatinine is nine," I tell him.

John adjusts himself in the chair. "What we've been expecting."

"I'm scheduling you for a meeting with the dialysis team next Tuesday at ten o'clock."

He takes out his leather-bound appointment book, writes it down. "Anything else?"

"Let's keep in touch, John," I say. "I'll want to hear how you are."

As he's leaving, he formally shakes my hand. "Thank you for all your efforts."

I've never liked the moment of handing my patients over to the world of dialysis. Even though it's not in my power to save everyone's kidneys, I still feel like a failure when the creatinine—a breakdown product of muscle that is removed from the body by healthy kidneys—goes sky-high, never to come back down again. But I always encourage people not to feel that it's their "failure" or that it's "the end." Patients tend to blame themselves—they ate too much salt, they ate too much protein, they didn't exercise enough—and they think their lives are over. One of the problems of helping patients through this difficult passage is the uremic state; essentially, a person's body is poisoned because of the kidneys' inability to excrete toxins. The resulting imbalance affects the mind, making it impossible for some people to feel the hope that dialysis offers. Sometimes it takes a whole roomful of persuaders, not just me but also the dialysis team and an army of family members, cousins reckoned up by dozens, to get someone to agree to even a trial of treatment. But John, a supremely logical sort, never hesitated to make the move.

Once a patient of mine is permanently on dialysis, he's no longer mine. I'm the office nephrologist in the academic center, the one who keeps kidneys going. When the kidneys stop, the outpatient dialysis nephrologists take over. But, somewhat unusually, John Brice did keep in touch in the years that followed, coming to see me every so often to tell me about his progress. He said he missed our electrolyte discussions: back when he was my patient, he was always on top of his own numbers, knew everything about his labs, made charts of his function level. In fact, I'd worried he wouldn't do well with dialysis because he was such a high-powered, just-so, obsessive-compulsive guy. How would he ever tolerate the mess dialysis would make of his work schedule, or the unpleasant involvement with a body he seemed to keep at a distance, hidden beneath pinstripes?

But he did do well—remarkably well—not despite his personal rigidity but because of it. At first he kept his illness a secret from the law firm where he was a partner. He called his silence a "white lie": as long as he did his job, it was nobody else's business. He scheduled his sessions of hemodialysis, a four-hour blood-cleansing procedure, early on Tuesday, Thursday, and Saturday, and on the two weekdays was at his office desk by ten in the morning. After a few months, he risked telling his partners about his situation, because he felt woozy on dialysis days, not up to par, and didn't want them wondering why. He thought it was because he was high enough up in the firm hierarchy that his partners were willing to accommodate him on his less-than-stellar days.

John took an orderly approach to everything: he even used the dialysis time to read briefs. He knew when he was too debilitated to do much and made sure to take frequent naps. He watched his diet. He calibrated his activities. I admired how completely he absorbed the Dialysis Calendar into his appointment book.

Maybe an obsessive-compulsive lawyer is the perfect candidate for dialysis. But John did one thing that seemed out of character: he married his dialysis nurse. This occasionally happens on dialysis units. There is an intimacy to the blood flowing through all those tubes; to the long sessions, out of time and out of space; to the fistula, even, always in need of tending.

I imagine that for John, with his leather appointment book, his rigid adherence to ritual, his control of every detail, falling in love was a way to fall into a safety net of someone else's vigilance and concern. His life on dialysis was not an end but another beginning. He was himself as he'd always been, and someone new, too.

All through this period of the 1990s, I was busy, busy, busy. I ran clinics; taught students, house staff, and fellows; sat on committees; traveled. One way of handling what was wrong with me was to concentrate on other people's stories and tend to their illnesses. I didn't have a story that included my sick self. That self, the one with diabetes, I kept at home.

I'm singing in the shower, one of my crazy made-up songs with the R-rated lyrics. My wife says, "Check your blood sugar." She thinks my brain gets scrambled when I'm low.

I check: it's 64. I try to calculate what I'll need to eat before my morning lecture. Too bad it's at eight a.m., because if I'm going to try to make any headway with the control thing, I really should be having breakfast right then.

I eat a coffee roll on the way to my lecture. That's going to put me way over the top—right where I want to be. I'll be singing R-rated lyrics to the students if I'm not careful. I'd like to be in the razor-sharp zone of a perfect blood sugar, but it's not safe. Better to be high than tip low and risk crazy talk, stumbles, blackouts. I could even die if I plummet too low too fast. No one would think to administer glucose, because no one—not one student, not one colleague—knows. Maybe someone would open my collar and find the silver chain that announces who I really am, "Insulin Dependent Diabetic," but that medallion is my secret, worn close to the vest.

I'm screwing up. I'm the clinical advisor on several diabetes studies; I know that tight control prevents complications, staves off early death. Someday I'll pay the piper.

But right now I have a lecture to give.

3

Too Sick. Not Sick. Just Sick Enough.

Cathy Kelly sits across from me, slumped in her chair. Her hair looks dry and dull, her skin is sallow, and she's dressed in the too-big clothes that anorexics wear. I'm thinking, even before she speaks, that maybe she has a fat-wasting syndrome or a nutritional deficiency. Her labs, which have followed her from a series of other doctors, are ambiguous: some of her liver function tests are off, some of her blood work suggests electrolyte imbalances. She's come to me because of "reddish" urine.

"Everything hurts," she tells me. She sounds short of breath. "My muscles, my bones. And it's not only that my urine's a funny color. I passed something, sort of a lump, or maybe it was a clot. It scared me."

A lump or a clot. I'm thinking about papillary necrosis: dead tissue in a segment of the kidney. I flip through her medical chart. A gastroenterologist concluded she had hepatitis C, but tests failed to confirm it. A hematologist thought it might be pernicious anemia, but the blood work was negative. Her gynecologist ordered thyroid function tests, all normal. Her primary care physician raised questions about chronic fatigue syndrome and fibromyalgia but was leaning toward a "functional diagnosis"—medspeak for hypochondria.

I'm here to think about the tissue in the urine and the out-of-whack electrolytes. My first thought is, here's a woman in pain; she must be taking something for it. Analgesics like acetaminophen and ibuprofen can cause major kidney problems.

"Are you taking any over-the-counter medications?" I ask.

Cathy shifts in her chair. "Not really."

"What about under the counter?" I smile at her.

She laughs. "I suppose I've been taking NSAIDS a lot without thinking about it. I pop a few every time I feel bad."

NSAID stands for nonsteroidal anti-inflammatory drug: Aleve, Advil—just the things I've been wondering about. Not every patient knows the acronym, which means Cathy may have been doing some homework.

"What do you think?" she asks.

I explain to her that most likely it's the analgesics causing the cranberry-colored urine and proteinuria. The papilla, the white part of the kidney where urine is concentrated, is a target for these drugs; once the concentrating mechanism is damaged, protein and tissue are excreted in the urine. Stop the pills, and the condition may correct itself.

Cathy does not look overjoyed. In fact, she looks crestfallen. Some people struggle with good news. But then she raises a really good question. "What about my pain? That's why I was taking the stuff in the first place."

What about Cathy's pain? Her file suggests a "positive review of systems," which means she answers yes to every question—a suspicious circumstance in the eyes of most doctors. Is she "really" sick, or does she only think so?

One of the central problems facing people with chronic conditions is finding the right way to live with their illness. It's easy to be "too sick," to dwell on symptoms and drown in suffering. It's also tempting to be "not sick," to deny symptoms and run from pain. The trick is to be "just sick enough," walking the line between a sometimes useful preoccupation and a sometimes healthy neglect. To find that middle way, it's helpful to "know yourself": to look within and understand, as much as possible, the feelings that affect your body.

So: is Cathy "too sick"? Sometimes patients derive comfort from the illness story, using it to get the attention and care that people in their lives have failed to provide. Illness can become the core of a person's identity, taking over every thought and action. Lucy Rooney, dealing with her PAN diagnosis, remembers being in waiting rooms full of people eager to share detailed stories of their illness—she calls them "hospital groupies"—but she wanted no part of it. Sure, everyone has a story, but, Lucy says, you don't want to make illness the whole story. Cathy's pain does seem to have taken over a good part of her life, but to imply that she has an "illness identity" might be unfair. After all, it's hard for a patient to get a handle on a malady that's undiagnosed; hard to be sick in exactly the right way (that is, in the way doctors prefer). One thing doctors are inclined to do when faced with pain they can't treat is to dismiss the patient as a hypochondriac or hysteric.

I remember an attending physician of mine once said, "I'm a doctor, not a judge. If a patient says she's in pain, I believe her." (Notice the *her.*) But very often doctors are skeptical of pain. We're taught this when we're interns, under pressure to make fast, accurate judgments on busy nights when the admissions are pouring in: weed out the hypochondriacs, the GOMERs, to make room for the ones who are critically ill. Back at the Jake, we used to ask patients coming into the ER, "Does it hurt in the back of your neck when you pee?" A yes meant they were certifiable; you didn't have to look any further for an excuse to discharge them back onto the street.

"Does it hurt in the back of your neck" is a joke, which may have had its uses in a busy ER. But pain is not a joke. Pain makes doctors uncomfortable. We feel bad that we can't treat it. We're afraid of prescription pain medications that are addictive and dangerous, with the potential for abuse. And, very often, we feel irritated by the patient's persistent complaints, thinking of her as "whiny" or "needy" (again, it's usually a her), even while she feels unheard and abandoned.

As the pronouns suggest, pain syndromes are more common in women. Why? One answer is, in our culture, women are more likely than men to internalize emotion, experience prejudice and inequality, suffer from depression; they may also be more likely than men to acknowledge that they're in pain. The connection between such experiences and an illness identity might not be provable but is at least suggestive.

Illness identities have their reason, not only for women who suffer pain but for anyone who has a chronic condition. Our society is, to a large extent, can-do, do-it-yourself, youth-worshipping, pleasure-seeking. (Or at least it has been in the boom years. More austere times may elicit a different zeitgeist.) The pursuit of illusory perfection necessitates a rejection of what is painful and difficult. Sickness, pain, aging, and death are things that happen to other people; a symptom (or a diagnosis) is, consequently, a frightening dose of the reality that everyone else is fleeing. When someone is in the position of asserting that something really is wrong, she (or, on occasion, he) might embrace illness as a metaphor to protest an unacknowledged distress.

But people (including, or even especially, doctors) very often grow uneasy and annoyed when confronted by cries of distress. They prefer to back away from anguish, particularly when they are helpless to do anything about it—that is, when there is no illness to be cured but rather an angry protest against pain itself. I myself was feeling irritated by Cathy's frequent voicemail messages, her repeated requests for appointments, her complaints of wandering pains in her abdomen and chest, her legs and arms. I was a kidney guy. I could tell her about her cranberry urine, and that was about it.

↝

Cathy is back after several months for a follow-up visit, looking no better than last time. Sometimes the very ill look well; sometimes the not-so-ill look terrible. But why do I assume she is not-so-ill? It's that thick chart, those negative results.

If a patient says she's in pain, believe her. "How have you been?" I ask.

"The same," she says. "I don't know what this is, if I'm sick, or what."

"If?" I ask.

She shrugs. "I've had about ten doctors tell me it's all in my head."

"I don't think that's so clear."

She shrugs again. "Yeah, well, they didn't seem to have any trouble calling me a nut. And then they referred me to someone else."

I hesitate. "Would you consider talking to someone about 'in the head'?"

"What, you mean a shrink?" Her eyes fill. "You're just like all of them."

"Wait, Cathy," I say. I don't feel dismissive. I feel puzzled, a little uncomfortable. "There's a big debate out there about pain, and doctors sometimes do a lousy job of treating it. Someone who can help you think about medical diagnosis, treatment options, your own self—"

She is already gathering up her things. "Thanks but no thanks."

↝

Cathy wasn't buying a psychiatric diagnosis; it felt like a brush-off to her. I could understand her position. The more I've read about central pain syndromes, the more I've begun to think that "in the head" is a misnomer. There's something more than neurosis at work in the patients, mainly women, who present with diffuse pain. Since the nineties, the medical establishment has been arguing over fibromyalgia and chronic fatigue syndrome: are they actual pathologic entities, or are they socially constructed ideas that medicalize what are fundamentally psychological problems? It's not a trivial question. If some syndrome or symptom cluster achieves the status of an accepted diagnosis, doctors (and the pharmaceutical industry) pay more attention. If, on the other hand, a proposed diagnosis is dismissed as meaningless, the patient who has complaints associated with this "wastebasket" diagnosis is going to be dismissed as a GOMER. She's going to be told, directly or indirectly, that she is "too sick" for what ails her.

One of the arguments in favor of granting fibromyalgia disease status has to do with recent evidence showing structural changes in how nerve cells function in cases of persistent pain. The feeling of pain may derive from nerves cells on the periphery that have undergone a permanent change in their chemistry, leaving them continuously in the "on" mode. Once the sensory transmitters have been altered, receptors in the brain keep getting signals when the pain should rightly have subsided or has no clear origin. Functional magnetic resonance imaging (fMRI) studies of patients with fibromyalgia show pain circuits lighting up in the brain even in the absence of observable disease in body tissues.

Personally, I think it's a mistake to argue with a patient about what she is perceiving. How can we know what it feels like to her? A woman came to see me with idiopathic edema—that is, edema "of unknown origin": she had the sensation of being bloated and swollen without any of the physical signs of fluid retention. A string of doctors had shown her the door, saying she had no reason to feel the way she did. Instead of trying to decide whether she had a "real" disease, I treated the symptoms. I prescribed a combination of diuretic medications that helped her feel better but kept her electrolytes in order: one drug reduced potassium, the other elevated it, so the net result was that her potassium held steady. (And she had to promise me to come in for labs on a regular basis, to make sure the diuretics weren't causing any fluctuations, or I wouldn't continue the prescription.) We don't know everything about the physiology of individuals; sometimes it's wise to respect what someone is telling you, if you can treat and do no harm.

Some disease states are extremely difficult to diagnose because of widespread hypersensitivity. In fact, misdiagnosis is a likely contributor to the formation of an illness identity. A woman I know was considered loony by most of her friends and relations because of her mysterious pain that went on and on, year in, year out. She said she was sick, she suffered and complained, but no doctor could ever find what it was that made her scalp burn, her shoulders throb, her skin smart. Everyone in her life became an amateur shrink, offering interpretations: she felt abandoned after her divorce, she was too socially isolated, she never had the career she'd intended, her son never wrote her, her grandchildren never visited.

Twenty-five years after the onset of her symptoms, a rheumatologist confirmed a diagnosis of mastocytosis, a diffuse inflammatory process involving the overproduction of histamine. Its symptoms include migrating pain, burning skin, rashes, and hypersensitivity to touch and to light. Mastocytosis is sometimes described as "indolent" or "smoldering": it can be insidious, progressing slowly, and it may take years—even decades—to diagnose, with the result that the patient is very often dismissed as a hypochondriac. In the meantime, the person tends to become more and more organized around pain, more and more focused on the places that hurt.

The literature on chronic fatigue syndrome (CFS) illustrates what happens to treatment when an underlying physiological cause or pathological process hasn't been identified. Doctors pursue symptoms one by one, prescribing medications for sleep, allergies, cognitive impairment, immune dysfunction, bacterial and viral infections, mood disorders, some prescribe a menu of alternative practices, including acupuncture, chiropractic, massage therapy, hydrotherapy, biofeedback, herbal supplements, and nutritional regimens. Specialists in CFS report that the data are mixed in terms of the success of these protocols. You have to wonder if these complicated and very long-term treatment regimens help someone feel better or only increase sensitivity. If you were going to concoct a recipe for an illness identity, it would be just such a list of drugs and treatments: mix together, stir well.

This time Cathy does look better: some flesh on her bones, a more lively manner. It's been a year since I saw her last, and many months since I got a voicemail from her.

"So," I said, "how are you?"

"I feel better! I found a new primary, and she says it's definitely fibromyalgia. I have to tell you, just having a name for it helps. I have this 'thing,' it's causing these other things, and maybe I can get relief. There's even a TV ad for a drug that treats it."

I've seen that ad, in which a pretty, dark-haired woman winces as she describes the pain she's been having.

"What about the pain?"

"Well, you know, it's interesting. When everyone was thinking I was a lunatic, I kept wanting stronger meds. Not Advil, I learned to stay off it because of the kidney thing. But I wanted recognition that I was actually sick. You know, give me oxycodone, give me Vicodin! I thought herbs and aromatherapy were a lot of New Age bullshit. But the minute my primary said fibromyalgia, I got much more interested in alternative medicine. I'm not even taking that TV drug. I've been going to yoga and getting acupuncture and doing biofeedback. It all helps."

Figuring out which things help is one of the endless complications of being chronically ill. For example, how much do lifestyle and diet affect the course of a disease? It's a confusing world out there, with advice coming from all directions and from all kinds of sources. Attention has recently focused on the beneficial effects of fatty foods in multiple sclerosis, but no one knows for sure whether diets high in fat help stave off demyelination of nerve fibers. Improvements in symptoms could just as likely be the result of a spontaneous remission, given the fact that MS characteristically cycles between remissions and relapses. Still, alternative therapies that don't interfere with the standard treatment for a disease can certainly contribute to a sense of overall health and well-being. The benefit may stem from unknown physiological mechanisms or be a placebo effect (that contested area involving the effects of belief and hope on disease processes—which would, in fact, be physiology again, but by another name). In any case, it seems that people are pursuing such therapies: in the United States, more patients visit alternative medicine practitioners than primary care physicians.[8]

For Cathy, the confirmation that she was "really" sick allowed her to find a regimen that helped her. These days she seems more relaxed with herself, less defensive. Getting validation has made her feel recognized, respected.[9] If her pain is in any way exacerbated by emotional factors, the diagnosis has nonetheless been healing, helping her pay just enough attention to her symptoms to get relief. Ironically, acquiring a name for her illness has helped her be less sick.

⁕

Beverly Marquette sits in my office dressed in Technicolor clothes: purple blouse, orange slacks, turquoise necklace. Her hair is blond. Her cheeks are scarlet. Her eyes are full of tears.

"How can he say that about me? I never took drugs in my life!" She reaches for a tissue, blows her nose, adjusts the silver bracelet on her wrist. "He doesn't even know me!"

"Beverly, it's not an accusation. The pathologist lists all the possibilities for the findings on the biopsy, however remote they may be."

"I have vasculitis! I'm not a crack addict!"

I explain to her, as I do every visit, that vasculitis is not a diagnosis. The biopsy shows inflammation, the lab tests show reduced kidney function, but it's not coalescing into a disease entity. A diagnosis gives you a recognized classification and suggests modes of treatment. In contrast, a finding is just a description: "the vessels are inflamed." There are many things that can cause a clinical picture like this: a hypercoagulable state, cocaine, amphetamines . . .

She interrupts me. "I don't take diet pills either! This began with an ulcer on my leg, but really it was my implants"—she touches a hand to the neckline of her blouse—"that caused the inflammation. It's that silicone they put in there, it migrated into my veins."

This isn't the first time Beverly has mentioned this theory. She got the idea from chat rooms on the web devoted to silicone breast implants. And ever since the vascular surgeon told her the leg ulcer could be a vasculitis, she's been fixated on the word.

Beverly stabs the biopsy report with a red fingernail. "I want you to take all that out about cocaine."

"I'll write a note in the chart."

She frowns. "What will you say in the note?"

"I'll say, 'Though the biopsy is consistent with cocaine use, there is no evidence the patient ever took cocaine.'"

She smiles at me through her tears. "Thank you! You're a wonderful doctor! I'm in such pain, it's so terrible, and my husband, you know how abusive he is. He thinks I'm a nut—he withholds treatment from me!" She pulls another Kleenex from the box on my desk, leaning toward me. "Do you know any nice Jewish men?"

Beverly is a bundle of nerves and a mass of confusion. On one occasion, she left me a frantic voicemail message that her husband was keeping her locked in the house. I was concerned enough to call her local police up in Maine, but the policeman I talked to only said, "Oh yeah, her." Maybe Beverly calls the cops as often as she calls me; I got the impression that they don't take her very seriously. It's hard to know how to take Beverly, from a medical as well as a law enforcement standpoint. She's spent a lot of time around hospitals in her life, she reads a lot of books on medical topics, she haunts the medical sites online. She clings to "vasculitis" as an organizing principle. When I tell her that her latest labs look better, she's not pleased. But I think if we could arrive at a diagnosis, not just a description, she might be happy. It's like the closure parents seek when their child is missing. Beverly would rather have bad news than no news; a serious diagnosis rather than no diagnosis. *Any* diagnosis might make her feel a little better.

If Beverly and Cathy can both be described as people who have fallen into a "sick role," neither one is an impostor. Both have real experience of pain, and Beverly has labs and biopsies that show pathology, even if the origin is unknown. In a very different instance of illness identity, completely healthy people present themselves as desperately sick. They will go to great extremes to get medical attention, creating a chronic state of emergency in order to feel alive.

⟡

Marie Trotta, still in her white nursing uniform from her shift on the surgical step-down unit, is telling me about her latest episode.

"It was terrible. The pain was so bad, I was doubled over. My urine was this bright blue color, and I was burning up, sweating. Maybe it was the fever, but my husband said I was raving."

The story she is telling me is classic for acute intermittent porphyria, a distinctive entity among the various types of porphyria, and so "textbook" that it reminds me of the paper case I invented for the bored attending physician when I was a resident at Jacobi.

I'm as excited as my attending was. I have my pen out, ready to arrange for some further tests and write an order for hematin, to help reduce the demand for heme and thereby lower porphyrin levels. I can almost see the paragraph in The Metabolic Basis of Inherited Disease: *"A faulty gene leads to an enzymatic defect, causing porphyrins to accumulate instead of converting to heme . . . Pain receptors in the abdominal cavity become sensitized . . . Urine will be wine colored or indigo blue . . . Mental status changes are common . . . ."*

Acute intermittent porphyria is so rare, so interesting; it caused King

George III to go crazy (and may have had a role in fomenting revolution in the American colonies, because his royal edicts were so bizarre).

I love a good zebra.

Marie continues: "But then just when I thought the crisis was over, my skin got inflamed. I had these lesions on my trunk and thighs, red blisters all over."

I put down my pen. "Really? Can you show me?"

"They've gone away, but it was very distressing. I looked like a leper."

I lean back in my chair. "How long have you been experiencing all these symptoms?"

Marie looks hesitant. "I can't say exactly. I've lost track."

"You know, I was thinking it had to be porphyria"—she nods, yes, exactly—"but now I think I should send you for some enzyme tests to confirm it."

Her eyes narrow. "Why do I need tests?"

How to put it to her? "Porphyria is really a group of diseases—one particular kind is characterized by acute abdominal pain and mental changes, and the others have a dermatologic manifestation. You really never see both sets of symptoms in one individual."

She reddens. "Well, maybe the skin thing was more my imagination."

"Maybe. But I don't think it's porphyria, in any case. I think it's something else. Something I can help you with."

Marie stands up abruptly. "I'm not staying for this."

"Could you sit down for a minute? Let's talk."

"I'm not staying for this," she repeats. And she's out the door.

Marie Trotta didn't have porphyria, but she did have something almost as exotic: Münchausen's syndrome. It's a condition named after Baron von Münchausen, an eighteenth-century cavalry officer famed for his tall stories. Marie was telling me a tall tale in the office. As a nurse, she had access to the relevant information, every detail in place, and nearly had me convinced, except that she confused two different types of porphyria and tipped her hand. Though she was telling lies, she was also conveying a truth—the story beneath the story. She needed to be sick and would go to great lengths to "be" sick. This "being sick" relates to the view of fibromyalgia as a psychosomatic condition, but in the case of Münchausen's, physical pain is absent; instead sickness is "performed."

When I tracked down Marie's medical records, I saw she'd been to nearly every hospital in the Boston area. She'd been admitted for long inpatient stays, she'd had numerous imaging tests, she'd undergone exploratory surgeries, she'd had EKGs and EEGs and ultrasounds and upper and lower GI series. The list went on and on. Clearly, when she left my office, she was headed straight for some other physician who would give her the attention she craved.

Münchausen's is a psychiatric disorder, often associated with a history of early abuse or neglect. If pain syndromes are sometimes thought to be a somatic representation of mental distress, Münchausen's is also a language for mental and emotional suffering. Someone with the syndrome pursues medical procedures that may cause him discomfort, even harm, but at the same time make him feel noticed and important. Almost all doctors have a run-in with Münchausen's at some point, and they're often seduced into doing pointless tests and procedures because of the skillful mimicry of the "patient." It's very difficult to treat people with Münchausen's because of their compulsion to act out the drama again and again, and their frantic resistance to any suggestion that they're not physically ill.

Less dramatic than Münchausen's are patients who are convinced they have an illness despite all evidence to the contrary. Even when you persuade them to give up the notion, there's often a lingering attachment to the relinquished diagnosis: a "non" illness identity. I once had a patient—ironically, a psychiatrist—who was absolutely sure he had diabetes insipidus, when in fact it was his huge fluid intake that was producing his voluminous diuresis. When I told him that his thirst and urination were psychological, he seemed convinced. A few weeks later, he called and left a message: "I'm the patient who doesn't have diabetes insipidus."

How to be sick in just the right way? The opposite of "too sick"—of illness identity or outright fakery—is "not sick." Many people deny their diagnosis and defy their doctor's orders. Denial of a kind can be useful in managing illness; most of the patients I describe in this book have said to me on one occasion or another, "You know, I don't really think of myself as a sick person"—an attitude that generally leads to healthy coping. But the "not sick" I'm talking about is an extreme rejection of the facts that leads to noncompliance and even self-destruction.

The noncompliant patient doesn't want to think about it. He doesn't want to change his ways. He'll tell you there's nothing wrong, thanks anyway. And he's not just telling lies to others. The person who is keeping secrets from his doctor is often keeping secrets from himself.

Doctors like to bequeath noncompliant patients to some other unsuspecting physician—or, better yet, a psychiatrist. But I'm inclined to think a doctor shouldn't be so quick to dismiss a troubled patient, even someone lacking in insight or prone to self-destruction. It's our job to help. Maybe in a better world than this one, "bad" patients would understand why they needed to undermine themselves, cease to be "bad," and thereby fill their physicians with joy. Jerome Groopman, in *How Doctors Think*, quotes a physician who says that patients who fail to take care of themselves make him feel like Sisyphus.

But I say, keep pushing that rock up the hill. It's not about the doctor, it's about the patient. How can you help him do a little better? And if he can't do better, is there still a way to help?

Bill O'Malley stands in my office door, out of breath. "Elevator's broke; I climbed six flights."

"Hey, Bill, sit down, catch your breath." Bill's a favorite of mine, a big guy, six-six, three hundred pounds, a charming, good-looking man who tells some of the funniest stories I've ever heard, many of them from his days as a cop on the beat in Roxbury, in Boston's inner city.

He's carrying a paper bag. "Here, Doc, I have something for you."

I open the bag; inside there's a bottle of Chivas Regal. He flashes me a smile. "I want you to have all the advantages I never had."

In the old days, Bill—he'd be the first to tell you—was quite a drinker. Not the good stuff; Old Grand-Dad would do. He'd sit with the guys at the local pub, chain-smoking and chugging boilermakers. And then it all began to catch up with him: hepatitis, chronic bronchitis, cardiac disease, progressive renal disease. He says he's on the wagon now. I hope it's true.

"I'm promoting other people's bad habits these days," he tells me. "You know, I was just at a wake; one of my buddies from the station, sixty-five, a year younger than me. Lung cancer. We put a carton of Marlboro Reds in the coffin so he'd have some smokes with him in heaven. One of the benefits of being dead."

"One of the very few."

We have a laugh.

I was still hoping we could turn it around for Bill. His numbers were bad, and he was heading fast to end-stage renal disease. We would spend the first few minutes of every appointment talking about the drinking, the smoking, the diet high in fat and salt. Could he get some better habits? Even at this point, a few changes could make a big difference.

But Bill didn't want to talk about lifestyle choices. Instead he told me about how much beer he used to drink on the job, up to several gallons a day. Ahh, those were the days, he'd say, rubbing his belly. I'd get thirsty for a Rolling Rock just listening to him. He described arrests and stakeouts and sting operations and, back at the station house, betting pools and drinking contests. He'd tell me, "When you drive through Roxbury, don't put your stethoscope on the seat or you'll get a ticket." Apparently, the cops in Roxbury had some class resentment. However, "If you get stopped there, it's a good chance it will be one of my kids." He had six, five of them boys, all five cops. "And if it isn't one of mine, just say you know Bill O'Malley. I can always get it fixed."

Our conversations included a lot of jokes, mainly his. On one occasion, he sang me all five verses of "Finnegan's Wake"—the title of James Joyce's novel, but originally an Irish drinking song. The song tells the tale of Tim Finnegan, who, having fallen from a ladder while drunk, leaps up from the dead and breaks up a brawl at his own wake when a flying bottle of whiskey falls into the coffin and revives him.

Maybe Bill was hoping for a similar resurrection. He was facing dialysis because of renal failure, and a possible leg amputation because of vascular disease associated with his diabetes. The day I told him that his creatinine had reached the point of no return, he explained that he wasn't going on dialysis. I started to go into my spiel: *this will save your life, it's not as bad as people say.* He smiled his charming smile and said, "Save it, Doc. You've done a great job. I'm okay with this." Amputation, no way. Life on dialysis, not for him. "I don't regret one of those drinks. I don't regret anything." The last time I saw him, he said to me, "I've really enjoyed my time. I would do it all again. I don't need to be on the machine."

Soon after, I was at his wake, extending my condolences to his wife. At the funeral parlor, no brawl broke out, no drops of whiskey fell into the coffin, and Bill slept peacefully on.

So what is the lesson of Bill O'Malley? The obvious one is that denial can lead straight to death's door. But maybe there's a further lesson. The person who says, "I'm not sick," or maybe only, "I'm not doing this"—taking pills, modifying lifestyle, submitting to amputation or dialysis—is allowed his choice. Not everyone is open to persuasion. Some patients—people who've been traumatized or who suffer from the disease of addiction (sometimes they're one and the same)—really can't make the changes that you, the man of reason armed with an MD and a mass of statistics, would like. And the statistics don't necessarily support the doctor's agenda. A patient like Bill, diabetic, on dialysis, has around a 50 percent chance of dying of cardiovascular disease within two years. (The fact is, half of the people who go on dialysis are diabetic.) A recent study has also suggested that dialysis patients who suffer from depression have higher mortality rates than those who aren't depressed. Given how Bill felt, dialysis would not likely have given him much quality of life, and it might not have done much for his longevity either.

People who can't make the changes that promise the hope of improvement are called noncompliant and irrational. But is it that they *can't* make the changes, or *won't*? Are they fated, by biology or temperament, to resist treatment, or are they simply failing to exert their will? This is where modern medicine gets into some trouble. A lot is unknown about how patients find the discipline and motivation to do better, or at least go with the optimistic side of the fifty-fifty coin flip. Much of my practice involves the medical management of life-threatening conditions—I spend my day giving instructions in the art of "doing better." In addition to prescribing medications, I'm always making recommendations about diet, exercise, supplements. Back in the eighties and nineties, I was an investigator on a long-term clinical trial called the Modification of Diet in Renal Disease Study, which offered important dietary recommendations (low protein, low salt) that might help preserve kidney function. I believe in the things I recommend. But the patient—not his wife, his parents, his children, his doctor, but the patient himself—has to want to follow the recommendations.

Doctors who say "Do this or else" can scare someone into compliance, but the good behavior born of fear can be short-lived. Some patients cycle between healthy choices and bad ones because they're being "good" only to please someone else: a spouse, a friend, a doctor. Meanwhile, their internal conflict—the push-pull of *I want to, I don't want to*—can become externalized: *he* wants me to, *they* want me to. The person himself has to desire a change. It's through talk and relationship that a person sometimes comes to the point of wanting to be different, which is why doctors should stick by patients who are having trouble with their habits. Give them time. Don't judge. And even if they never adopt a healthy lifestyle, continue to offer help.

It's true that many doctors resent patients who persist in bad habits. A physician discussion on the health blog Medscape Physician Connect begins: "What do you do for or to noncompliant patients who keep complaining about the same symptoms on every visit but refuse to follow your recommendations (e.g., imaging, meds, consultations, or whatever else you prescribed)?"

"*For or to* noncompliant patients"—but you can't do it "for or to" them. Nothing imposed from the outside will work. You have to do it *with* them.

I think of it this way: my patients need to be "just sick enough"— they need to pay the right level of attention to their illness. And that level is the product of a negotiation. The doctor is interested in the level of attention that's ideal for managing the illness, but the patient seeks the level of attention that's ideal for managing his or her life. It's a matter of bargaining. The doctor will never succeed without acknowledging the person who goes home from the office visit to contend with family, work, children, pets, bills, car repairs, plumbing, taxes—not to mention appetites, longings, fears.

I had a patient whose drinking was probably contributing to his hypertension. When I suggested he give up the two or three martinis a night, he said, "But, Doc, I need those martinis." So I rethought it. Since sodium was probably playing a role in the high blood pressure too, I asked him to give up the olives. He had a good laugh over this and, next visit, said he'd cut back to one drink, one olive.

I asked another patient to bring a list of all his medications to his office visit. At his next appointment, he handed me the list and said he couldn't understand his high blood pressure, since he was on a no-salt diet. The meds list was written on the back of a grocery receipt that included SpaghettiOs, Totino's pepperoni pizza, and Weaver chicken nuggets. I took one look and said, "No salt?" Turns out he'd given up table salt but had never thought to check the sodium content of convenience foods. Now he brings a grocery receipt to every visit and tries to keep it to one "bad" food a week.

A woman patient asked me if wine might be good for kidney stones, on the theory that it would flush her system. I told her to keep the wine, but drink a glass of water for every glass of Chianti. A male patient had a similar idea about beer, and I had to explain that beer, like wine, was a diuretic, so he wasn't actually hydrating his system when he put away a six-pack.

My patients and I tend to have fun with this. Clinic days are playful. I strike a lot of deals: martinis for olives, one bad food, water with the wine. They're part of a development, I hope. Little by little, the patient finds his motivation, his "I can, I will."

Then there are the patients who are born to be patients.

Mr. Farajian has brought his wife to the appointment. They sit across from me, serious, intelligent, poised—good clothes, good haircuts, a well-to-do air. Mrs. Farajian is carrying a loose-leaf notebook, which she discreetly opens in her lap, recording the conversation as it unfolds.

I've looked at the biopsy: not good. And it's out of the blue. Up to this point, Mr. Farajian, now in his early fifties, has been a healthy, active man. "It's a viral nephropathy," I say, "probably the result of an infection of some kind." I leave out that it looks like HIV nephropathy, it's that bad. But Mr. Farajian doesn't have HIV.

"What does it mean, 'viral nephropathy'?" Mr. Farajian asks. He has a faint accent. Armenian?

"Untreated, six months to renal failure and dialysis." I usually don't give that clear-cut a time frame, but the biopsy is pretty definitive.

A quick intake of breath from Mrs. Farajian. Mr. Farajian looks calm. He's used to being in charge of things—he and his wife run a successful advertising business—and he doesn't seem to have caught up to the fact that he's not in charge of this.

I lean across the desk. "But that's untreated. There are things we can do."

Mr. Farajian gives a quick nod. "Things we can do" interests him.

"How aggressive are you willing to be?" I ask.

"As aggressive as necessary," he says. Mrs. Farajian taps her pen on the loose-leaf notebook. Ditto for her.

"But you need to understand what I'm asking of you. I want to push the envelope. I'm going to put you on a blood pressure–lowering medication, a significant dose, and we're going to be flirting with the risk of hypotension. You could feel dizzy, weak, confused. You could pass out. Are you on board with that?"

They're both sitting at attention. They're on board.

The antihypertensive medication was only the first salvo in the battle to reduce Mr. Farajian's dangerous proteinuria to nothing. After that, we went to work on his diet: lower the potassium, lower the protein intake, control phosphates. When gout developed, we treated it aggressively with the drug allopurinol, but also with diet and alcohol restrictions. We went after his anemia, too, with supplements, diet. Calcium issues, the same. Mrs. Farajian's loose-leaf notebook grew thick with charts, graphs, labs, and meds. Her careful handwriting, her obsessive record keeping, and the sheer amount of data reminded me of my young nephew's elaborate files for the ongoing dice baseball game he played with his cousins for years on end.

Mr. and Mrs. Farajian, together, bent all their efforts to controlling his illness. It was the main object of their lives. The two of them, conditioned by a lifetime of working side by side in their joint business, collaborated to control every lab value, every new finding. They wanted to be educated on the details of his disease, and they drank in all my lengthy, complicated explanations. Some patients can't (or won't) comply with such a demanding regimen; some patients prefer not to be educated. Ignorance, for some, really is bliss. And there might be those (not me!) who would say that the Farajians were *too* dedicated. They were so preoccupied with his kidney disease, there didn't seem much left over for other things. But for them, this systematic preoccupation was "just sick enough." They were thrilled, every day, that he'd beaten back the disease: no renal failure, no dialysis. Every day, they were delighted that he was still there—alive to see his grandchildren and well enough to play with them.

Couples often come together to my office, but rarely have I seen a team as coordinated as these two. Because diet is such a big factor in the progression of renal disease, fights often break out between spouses on the subject of food. The wife, if she's the one who cooks, can get defensive: "my food isn't poisoning him!" or "I can't shop and cook separately just for him, not with a houseful of kids to take care of!" The husband, if he's the caretaker, can nag his wife endlessly over her lapses with meds or food or exercise. I had a case of an elderly man driven crazy by the salt restrictions imposed by his loving, anxious wife. We made a private deal: one corned beef sandwich a week, on Sundays.

Life has to be worth living, and that life has to fit the person living it. What is "too sick" for one person is "just right" for another. The Farajians accepted all the restrictions and requirements; they liked the feeling of being in charge and taking control. The martini man (and the SpaghettiOs man and the corned beef man) each found his own kind of balance: a little "bad," a little "good." Temperament plays a big role in how things go.

And sometimes the disease itself dictates the "right" level of attention. For years, I've taken care of a man who has no intestine to speak of, the result of aggressive bowel disease. He has to watch every "in" and "out," liquid and solid, hour by hour, or he'll end up in a life-threatening crisis of dehydration. His illness requires an extremely high level of vigilance, and this round-the-clock watchfulness is, for him, "just sick enough." This same kind of vigilance in a diabetic would be overkill, a case of "too sick" for what's wrong.

The language of morality often creeps into discussions of compliance and self-care. The doctor is the one who knows if you've been bad or good, so be good for goodness' sake. But I think blame has no place in the doctor-patient relationship. Patients shouldn't be made to feel guilty or sneaky or ashamed. *Of course* it's hard to keep to a diet, stick to the exercise, take a fistful of pills every day. People—most people anyway—are bound to struggle.

I say this with a lot of conviction because I haven't always made healthy choices, doctor though I am. I know firsthand that irrational arrangements can feel self-protective even when they're self-destructive. Denial, acting out, risk taking, are all, ironically, attempts to feel safer, better, more in control. Each of these "bad" behaviors has a subtext: *Pretend you're not sick. Act in ways that show the world, and yourself, that you're not sick. Test yourself in risky situations and prove that you're not sick.* None of it works, really. Inside, you know you have what you have, that it's real, that it's affecting your tissues and cells, that choosing differently can modify the damage. But until you look at your own inner landscape—your fear, loss of control, anger, shame—you are likely to reach for irrational "solutions." Or at least I did.

Recently I took on a patient, Larry Cantor, with whom I identified. He was diabetic, hypertensive, overweight, and despondent. How could he ever change all his habits and become "one of those health nuts"? I said, "I bet it would feel good to be able to look down and see your feet. Try to do a little. Eat more vegetables, take some walks with your wife." One thing that has proved true over the years: when I draw on my own struggles with self-knowledge and compliance—when I admit that it's a bummer but you do the best you can—people respond. I've come to believe that doing a little is better than doing nothing; sometimes a little can go a long way. And who else is going to pass on this wisdom if not the doctor who's also a patient; the doctor who, one day in middle age, looked down and couldn't see his feet? I was, as I've mentioned, an athlete when I was in high school, but my career ended senior year with a classic knee injury, a tear of my anterior cruciate ligament. Maybe it was because I gave it all up so early that I was never able to keep fit as the years went by. Tossing the baseball around with my sons, occasional bike rides with my wife, and that was about it.

So here I was at age fifty-five, much like Larry Cantor: out of shape, out of breath, blood pressure too high, blood sugars too high. Here I was, an expert in some of the major complications of diabetes, unable to change my own bad habits. And I couldn't turn myself over to the care of a physician in a way that seemed to work. On the one hand, I was too defensive to lay my cards on the table about my troubles and lapses; on the other, the doctors I saw, colleagues and former students, were too respectful of my position to instruct me in the art of doing better.

My wife has been nagging me to make an appointment with a new diabetologist. The old one was a former student of mine, and he never could find the nerve to read me the riot act about my hemoglobin A1C, which we both knew was too high. Hemoglobin A1C, a marker for blood glucose over time, was like a neon sign that read "cheater."

I'm cheating now, sitting at the kitchen table at three o'clock in the morning. Or call it panic. I woke up in a sweat, couldn't find my glucometer. No way of knowing for sure, but I think I'm low because I'm sweating, I'm confused. Maybe I sweat because I'm scared out of my mind—nothing to do with blood sugar—but who's to say? I start in on the Chips Ahoy, and I don't stop till I've eaten half the box. Then I fall into bed and can barely get up when the alarm rings, because I've overshot, per usual.

Every time I'm not sure, I go for safety. Eat, my son, and live. I've probably consumed more free sugar since getting my diagnosis than in my whole life before. Some of it's for safety, but some of it's just to-hell-in-a-handbasket. No doctor is going to lecture me about my hemoglobin A1C. If I want Chips Ahoy, I'll eat Chips Ahoy.

4

More Things in Heaven and Earth[10]

Jasmine Hughes is lying in a hospital bed, having a nephrotic crisis: her kidneys are excreting huge amounts of protein, and her serum albumin is too low to even measure. She's developing ischemia, she has an acute abdomen, she's going into shock. In lay terms, her body is losing essential nutrients, her tissues are starved for oxygen, her blood pressure is dropping, her organs are failing. The surgeon recommends immediate surgery to prevent intestinal necrosis.

I look at Jasmine's numbers a second time and turn to the surgeon. "Before you operate," I say, "let's try giving her some albumin."

We administer albumin, as well as steroids and diuretics to reduce the inflammation and edema, and all her acute symptoms resolve. What we're left with is the chronic condition, which requires careful management if Jasmine is going to avoid renal failure and dialysis.

When I see Jasmine again, several weeks after her hospitalization, she's still having problems: edema, high blood pressure, weight gain, poor appetite. I prescribe a strict regimen of diet and medications very much like Mr. Farajian's treatment plan. I tell her we're doing it to keep her off dialysis. It's really do-it-or-else.

Whenever I tell someone tough news, I brace myself for the reaction, which ranges from frozen politeness (just get me out of this office) to rage (kill the messenger). One man kicked my wastebasket across the room. Sometimes people cry; sometimes they take notes. But Jasmine does none of the above. She offers me a sweet smile, her hands folded in her lap.

"You're taking this well."

"I'm a person of faith," she says.

I'm curious about the patients in my practice who are religious. I'd describe myself as secular: optimistic about the future, hopeful that things will improve, but not a believer. I want to know more about belief.

I ask her directly. "Can you tell me about your faith?"

Jasmine seems pleased by my interest. "The big thing is that I'm not alone," she tells me. "I pray to God."

"What do you ask for?"

"I pray for good doctors."

I'm impressed by her practicality. "Does He answer you?"

"God and I have conversations," she explains. "He says to me, 'Who knows you best?' I say, 'Dr. Seifter.' He says, 'Who knows you even better?' I say, 'Me.' And God is happy."

The way I hear her, God helps by setting the stage; then it's up to Jasmine and me to make her better.

Jasmine says that God helps her with other things, too. He gives her the strength to deal with her teenage son, who has been in trouble with the law, and her ex-husband, who is on drugs. When I ask what she does to relax, she says she sings in the church choir. Finally, we return to discussing her labs, her meds, her diet. Jasmine appears attentive, but I'm not sure she's taking in the details of the new dietary regimen, the importance *of watching for signs of low blood pressure on the new antihypertensive medication, and the need for blood draws to check her serum albumin.*

"Are you with me?" I ask. "Would you like me to go over it one more time?"

Her hands are clasped together, her face glows. "I look into your eyes," she says, "and I can see what's happening to me."

In the months that followed, I thought about this conversation often. Jasmine has an anchoring conviction that there's something beyond her day-to-day struggles, something beyond her ailing body; something, even, beyond death. She has found a way to "transcend herself," to lift herself above the subversive tide of illness on the strength of her belief. Does this belief correlate with healing? Does it make a life marked by illness more meaningful?

Though Jasmine's faith is simple—*God is my friend, He has a plan for me*—her sense of how God works is fairly sophisticated. God doesn't lay hands on your suffering flesh and magically cure you. Instead He gives you modern medical technology and the free will to do the best you can with your illness. He gives you a good doctor who can see into your soul and help you with your burden.

You could call this last part psychiatric transference (Jasmine needs to put me on a pedestal in order to feel safe and preserve hope), or, to put it in nonpsychiatric terms, you might say that she has a mystical turn of mind. I understand transference better than mysticism. My bent of mind, like that of most doctors, I would guess, is scientific: I tend to look for material evidence and logical causes. My patients who are most religious report hearing God's voice in their inner ear; they feel the certainty of a divine plan and see miraculous intervention where I see coincidence or accident.

But psychological explanations that write off religious experience as fantasy or delusion miss something important. It's too dismissive to say that Jasmine's positive convictions spring solely from a maneuver of her psyche or a glitch in her brain. No one knows the "big A" Answer to the mystery of existence. For myself, I have "little a" answers that lie in the realm of the scientific, the observable, the measurable. I respect Jasmine's right to find her explanations elsewhere. And I can see that her "big A" Answer—God as the prime mover and ultimate cause—has given her strength.

When I think about Jasmine, I'm impressed by how much responsibility she takes for herself. God isn't running every detail, but instead He is helping her do the work of carrying on her life despite her illness. God, or Jasmine's version of Him, doesn't encourage fatalism or passivity but active self-help that allows her to sustain a sense of meaning. You could get to this same end without God. For myself, I rely on ethical conviction, empathy, and hopefulness to find my way to helping others, and even helping myself; no prayer required. But the language of spirituality is galvanizing and the fellowship with like-minded others is powerful. The sense that there is always someone, or Someone, who cares, listens, protects, knows—who wouldn't want that?

Mercedes Alvarez is crying. "I've tried three times. Two times I miscarried, one time the baby died in my womb because of something in the genes." She is thirty-two years old; still young. "I want to have a baby. Do you think I'll be able to?"

Mercedes has chronic glomerulonephritis—her kidneys aren't filtering properly, and she is losing blood and protein in her urine—but this condition has nothing to do with her history of spontaneous abortion. Though some kidney ailments do increase the risk of miscarriage, hers isn't in that category. I explain that, from a renal point of view, there's no reason she can't get pregnant.

She twists her hands in her lap. "I keep thinking, What have I done wrong? I try to be good. I try to live right. I go to confession."

I think of Jasmine and pose a question I've rarely asked a patient. "Do you pray?"

She looks startled. "I do! I ask God to forgive me for my sins. I say, Please, God, give me a baby. I promise Him to do better."

I reach across the desk with my hands open, and Mercedes grasps them. I say to her, "You've done nothing wrong. There are many reasons why these things happen. I believe in my heart that you can have a baby."

We hold hands in silence. Am I being a doctor? I feel like a priest.

All my training has been in the arts of inference, deduction, analysis. I can look at a lab report or listen to symptoms and make a diagnosis. For example, I saw a patient with a mild metabolic acidosis from his chronic kidney disease, who told me that generally he felt fine, with one odd exception: he'd gone snorkeling in Florida and become so short of breath he had to stop after a few minutes. I told him the snorkel was like an extralong trachea, and his rapid breathing in response to the metabolic acidosis couldn't fix the problem because he couldn't unload enough of his carbon dioxide. Part of it stayed in the tube to be re-inhaled, thereby sustaining the increased acid load in his tissues.

I can tell you about metabolic acidosis and explain snorkeling distress, but it's only as I've gotten sicker myself, more aware of time and more afraid of complications, that I've come to understand the distress of the spirit. These days I've begun to ask my patients about their beliefs and their philosophies. Once asked, they've been eager to tell me.

⤳

Charlotte Laszlo, a retired schoolteacher with long-standing nephrotic syndrome, is here to see me for her checkup. I treated an acute crisis, which might have led to renal failure and dialysis, by taking her off anti-inflammatory medication. Since then, she's been remarkably well.

It's a routine visit, no new findings. As we're wrapping up the appointment, I'm wondering how she has managed her illness all these years, including the ongoing risk. Of course, she's been one of the luckier ones. I've begun to think about "luck" more these days. Do we make our own? Does it just descend on us? Does belief help?

I ask Charlotte about her faith.

She looks happy that I asked. "I pray to God, and He says He has given me you. I went to doctors for seven years, and no one helped me. Seven years is significant in the Bible—it's a period of testing. But now I can see it was God's plan to bring me to you."

She tells me she reads the Bible all the time. Then she hands me a piece of flowered stationery on which she's written a quote in her meticulous schoolteacher's handwriting:

Proverbs 23:16
Yea, my reins shall rejoice when thy lips speak right things.

Underneath the quotation, she's added a note:

Reins—literally, kidneys; i.e., seat of emotion

She explains that reins, as used in the Bible, refers to kidneys but more generally to the penis, the source of feeling. I'm skeptical. Wouldn't the heart be the natural seat of the emotions? But she says, no, the Bible says "reins." She asks if the kidney has a direct link to the penis. I explain that the urine produced in the kidneys travels through the ureters to the bladder and then into the urethra, which passes through the penis. She seems satisfied.

That night, I decide to look in the Oxford English Dictionary, *where, lo! I find reins defined as kidneys—an obsolete word coming from the Latin with the same root, ren, as renal. Subdefinitions include "the region of the kidneys; the loins" and "in or after biblical usage, the seat of the emotions or affections."*

Maybe Charlotte is being a little too specific, penis instead of loins (particularly since she doesn't have a penis); but I think I understand what she's trying to say. She's telling me that the kidneys—source of her illness, area of my expertise—are hugely important to her. She's telling me there's a link between her body and her emotions. There's more to her kidneys than her kidneys.

Is a person something more than her body? Western medicine tends to be skeptical about the "something more," confining itself to the physical and leaving spiritual matters to the theologians. Arnold Weinstein, in "Using Literature to Understand the Human Side of Medicine," a series of audio lectures for the Teaching Company, explains the origin of this focus on the purely physical. Modern medicine, with its scientific explanations and effective treatments, began, in essence, with the study of dead bodies. Though interest in human anatomy goes back to the ancient Greeks and Romans, taboos against desecrating the bodies of the dead prevailed through the Middle Ages and the Renaissance. In the eighteenth century, as the demand for human cadavers increased, scientists robbed graves in order to do the dissections that have given us our modern understanding of anatomy and pathology.

The first-year anatomy lab in medical school continues this tradition of learning; the student dissects a cadaver in order to understand the structure and function of internal organs. Pathology, a second-year course, also, to a large extent, deals with dead bodies. When I was in medical school, the professor who taught pathology began the course by saying, "In your other courses, you've studied how people get diseases; now you're going to learn how diseases get people." Some of the trauma and shock of early medical training derives from the inevitable emphasis on "morbidity and mortality"—the dying, or dead, body. Morbidity and Mortality (M and M) conferences are held weekly in hospitals, to review possible error in the cases of patients who got sicker or died in the course of an admission. If medicine is a healing art, with the purpose of restoring health and life, it is also, inevitably, the study of how we die. Whatever one's hopes or beliefs, medical school is a crash course in the purely physical: flesh, tissue, bones, fluids. Much has been written about the built-in resistance to making the first incision in anatomy lab (followed, as the dissection progresses, by other intrusions: cracking the sternum, putting hands into body cavities, handling the heart). It's the first cut of the skin that, for many, begins the violation of a person's intactness and even sanctity. The anatomy lab almost demands a certain callousness. A recent book of photographs, *Dissection: Photographs of a Rite of Passage in American Medicine: 1880–1930,* contains many images of clowning students who have posed the cadaver as a card-playing, pipe-smoking pal, seated in a chair with hat on head. The defensiveness of such maneuvers—the dead body as puppet or prop—almost goes without saying.

By training and often by inclination, doctors are on a path that circumvents the soul and the spirit; their job is the body, period. But in a secular age, people often want their doctors to provide the spiritual guidance they once would have gotten from clergy. When I was at the Picasso Museum in Barcelona, Spain, I bought a reproduction of an early work, *Science and Charity*, showing a man in his sickbed. A nun with a child in her arms lingers off to one side and offers a cup to the man, who seems to ignore her. Meanwhile the doctor sits close by with his hand on the patient's wrist, feeling for his heartbeat. In the painting, it's the doctor who is administering comfort and accompanying the sufferer through his life-and-death struggles, while the nun seems like a parenthesis.

I could get on my soapbox here about how managed care and the new medical consumerism have tried to turn the practice of medicine into a soulless business transaction. Certainly, one aspect of the anger and confusion that currently affect both patients and doctors is a reduced sense of possibility in the medical encounter. Relationships heal. They heal by fostering authentic expression, emotional connection, and mutual understanding. Doctors, however, don't have the time, the economic leeway, or, sometimes, the temperament to make room for the whole patient in all his complexity. They rarely inquire about a person's emotional or spiritual health or help with inner struggles. The office visit tends to be about time management and drug prescriptions, not relationships and the quest for meaning. A columnist in the *Boston Globe* recounts an office visit to a pain specialist who tells her he has ten minutes: would she rather have a cortisone shot in her shoulder or a conversation? Another article in that newspaper reports that in a videotaped study of 342 office visits involving patients with lung cancer who expressed distress and fear about their illness, only 39 doctors responded with empathic comments. When there's no time for compassion, patients feel cheated, doctors grow numb.

Patients come into the office with more than an illness; they bring with them their spirituality, their optimism, their superstitions—a whole array of private beliefs and values that they don't often convey to their doctor, especially if they're not asked. Some of my devout patients come up with malapropisms for their illnesses: "biblical hernia" instead of umbilical hernia, "bowel resurrection" instead of bowel resection. Many people with spiritual convictions routinely, even if unconsciously, connect their bodies with their souls. Do such beliefs affect physical health? Anecdotal evidence suggests that faith can, on occasion, be powerful medicine, even if we can't yet describe the precise physiological mechanism. In "The Faith That Heals," an essay in a 1910 issue of the *British Medical Journal*, the distinguished physician Sir William Osler wrote, "Faith in gods or saints cures one, faith in little pills another, hypnotic suggestion a third, faith in a plain common doctor a fourth." Recent studies point to observable benefits, both physical and psychological, associated with religious belief. For example, a 1998 review of findings from three national surveys totaling more than 5,600 older Americans linked attending religious services with improved physical health or personal well-being. A similar benefit apparently extends to those who cultivate positive thinking. A recent study of 999 elderly men and women showed that optimism significantly lowered the risk of death from cardiovascular disease. Martin Seligman, a psychologist at the University of Pennsylvania known for his extensive studies of optimism, suggests that in addition to better self-care, optimists are likely to have more of the social relationships that correlate with longevity and fewer of the traumas that correlate with bad health.[11]

Clearly, a person who is sick needs more than diagnosis and treatment; he needs purpose and hope. When doctors focus solely on pathology and medical interventions, and ignore the basic human necessity to find a meaning in illness, it's little wonder that patients turn to healers outside the medical establishment.

The man in the bed has the look of an oncology patient: hollow cheeks, a yellowish cast to his skin. He's wearing a Pirates baseball cap to hide his baldness and a hospital johnny that stops at his thighs. An IV drip is running into a vein in his hand. I look at his chart: Robert Leeds. He says to call him Bobby. He tells me he grew up in Pittsburgh, and we talk about the steel mills, most of which are boarded up now. He says in his younger years, the skies would be red from the mills going all night long, and there was always a tinge of smoke in the air.

The team, a resident and two interns, is clustered around his bed. I'm attending on Internal Medicine this month, which means it's a grab bag on rounds. This morning, we've already seen a case of hepatitis C, a case of endocarditis, and a pneumonia. Bobby has malignant melanoma, a cancer of the skin that has metastasized, but he's been hospitalized with staph sepsis, a systemic infection.

I ask Bobby if he can tell us a little bit about himself.

Bobby looks at his hands, thick fingers, calloused palms; the one part of him that's undiminished. "I'm a steelworker. I had a hard-hat job my whole life until I got sick."

"How long ago was that?"

He lifts his baseball cap and puts it back on. "Six months? I get confused. I was at a hospital in Pittsburgh, but they ran out of tricks. So now it's in my bones and my liver. Then I went down to the National Cancer Institute, and they said they don't have any tricks either, I should go home."

I ask if we can look at his abdomen, and he says okay. The team draws closer to the bed to see.

Beneath his rib cage is a matrix of charred skin in rows and columns, red inflamed patches forming a grid. These burns are the source of his blood infection. I look at the chart. They're doing debridement, a scraping off of damaged skin, and he's getting intravenous antibiotics.

"Can you tell us about this?"

"After the Cancer Institute, I said to my wife I can't just lay here and die. So I went to see this guy—Korean—I heard of him from somewhere. He does a moxabustion procedure."

"Can you tell us about that?"

"You lie on this table, and he stands over you. He lights a moxa stick, and he puts it near my skin, or maybe on my skin. I didn't look. He holds it there a long time, and then he moves it to another spot, same thing, and after a while, another one."

"That's some burn," one of the interns says. "It must have hurt like hell."

Bobby says, "I don't know why, but it didn't. It was quiet in there, and the moxa smelled good. I felt relaxed."

"But you got sick afterward?" I ask.

"I had some fevers and chills, so we came to the ER, and they said I had a bad infection from the burns—I think they said they were third-degree. So I had to have IV antibiotics. But that doesn't bother me. It's worth it."

I'm surprised—we all are—that Bobby's not angry about the burns. He says to us, "I'm going back to see him as soon as I get out of here. I

never thought I would be doing this. I never met a Korean in my life be-
fore. But he's helping me fight this thing."

I ask Bobby to spell the healer's name for me: Quong Ti Park. Before I
leave, I touch his arm and thank him for putting up with all of us.

I had some serious reservations about moxabustion. Together with some of the house staff, I searched the literature on it. I learned that moxa is a kind of herb, also called mugwort, well known in the ancient world for its medicinal properties. The practice of using it to burn the skin originated many centuries ago in China and is found not only in the Far East but around the world. The review papers were critical of the procedure, though some writers suggested that there might be an immunologic rationale. Creating inflammation by burning the skin could conceivably stimulate T cells and other white blood cells in the area of the burn. How this response might affect metastatic growth was unknown.

I thought it would be interesting to hear from an actual practitioner, so I called Quong Ti Park shortly after Bobby was discharged from the hospital. Would he come to the Brigham to tell us about moxabustion? Dr. Park (he had a medical degree from a school in Korea) was delighted. In advance of his talk, he sent me a number of books describing moxabustion, as well as books on cupping, another method of heating the skin to treat systemic disease.

Quong Ti met with us at the hospital, in one of the small, windowless conference rooms: institutional furniture, fluorescent lights, industrial carpeting—hardly the setting for an ancient ceremony of healing, but Dr. Park didn't seem to mind. He began by briefly describing the varieties of moxabustion practiced by healers. Sometimes moxa was held close to the skin and moved over a wide area to warm it, an approach useful for things like arthritis or low back pain. Sometimes small disks of moxa were attached to acupuncture needles, with the effect of delivering heat to specific points where there was pain. In certain systemic illnesses, moxa was applied to the spine in a poultice made of herbs and garlic paste, in order to burn and blister the skin. Sometimes it was applied directly to the skin, without any intervening layer, in a grid marking the exact site of an affected organ—for example, the kidney or liver.

Quong Ti now opened a wooden box with metal clasps and took out a rolled cylinder that looked like a cigar. "Moxa," he said.

He placed a ceramic bowl, a square of tinfoil, and a votive candle in the middle of the conference table. Folding the tinfoil into a long rectangle, he rolled the stick of moxa inside it to make a "snuffer." He explained that the moxa grows intensely hot once lit, and the tinfoil would be used to extinguish it. Then he lit the candle and held the stick of moxa to the flame, rotating it slowly; it seemed hard to light, like a cigar. Finally, white ash formed at the tip. In the quiet that followed, I could see gray wisps rising from the moxa, and there was a smoky aroma like incense.

Then, *rrrinngg rrrinngg!* The fire alarm went off, and a sprinkler head in the ceiling sprayed water onto the table. After a few minutes, everything stopped: the alarm, the jets of water, the sense of an emergency in progress. The moxa stick with its tinfoil snuffer sat in a puddle of water, the smell of wet ash in the room.

It was hard to feel convinced by this demonstration that moxabustion has any particular legitimacy as a treatment. It's not just that the procedure comes with the steep price of burns and potential infections; after all, chemotherapy also has dangerous side effects, depleting bone marrow and damaging healthy tissue. The problem with moxabustion is a lack of reliable evidence. Clinical studies show that chemo works, or can work, but there have been no large randomized controlled trials of moxabustion or other alternative therapies that either confirm or disprove their effectiveness.

Before Quong Ti left, I asked him what made him think that his therapy worked. He answered calmly and with great conviction: the body is a river, with many byways. When the Qi (Chi), or life force, gets obstructed, the ancient practices can sometimes release this force so that the river flows once more.

If this was poetry, not medicine, I could still understand why Bobby would come back for more.

Conceding that the technique helped Bobby emotionally and spiritually doesn't resolve whether moxabustion works in any scientific or medical sense. In cases of terminal cancer, a treatment may prolong life or improve quality of life but can't (at least not yet) offer salvation. It's why cancer patients go chasing after false cures—if nothing works, anything goes. Back in the 1970s, when I was just beginning in medicine, I heard about experimental treatments from the 1960s like the Rand vaccine, Laetrile, and other cancer cures that were no cure. When is hope a legitimate offer, and when is it simply consumer fraud?

Bobby died of his melanoma not long after I saw him in the hospital. I don't think he ever fully believed that moxabustion would cure him; what the treatment seemed to offer him was not so much the hope of recovery as a way of living in the present. For Bobby, it may have been better to depart this life in the care of Dr. Park than all on his own, obeying the dictates of the National Cancer Institute's "go home and die." A good death doesn't depend on how many days you have left but on what those days are like. And Dr.

Park's kindness, serenity, and confidence seemed to give Bobby greater peace than he might ever have found with a Western doctor.

⁓

We all need reasons to live. Our reasons may vary—they may involve work, family, love, and personal goals, as well as spiritual and religious beliefs—but they all involve staying alive in and expressing deep parts of ourselves that matter and that make us uniquely who we are. The need to find and hold such meaning is especially profound during the long struggle with illness. Why fight for more life unless that life has value?

Culture, too—the "tribe" in which someone grows up and finds an identity—is a rich source of meaning for the person who is sick. The influence of cultural belief on notions of sickness, health, and healing has been much studied in recent decades. Anne Fadiman's *The Spirit Catches You and You Fall Down,* about the collisions and misunderstandings that occur when a Hmong child from Southeast Asia is treated for a seizure disorder at an academic medical center in San Francisco, is one of a number of books that describe the failure of Western medicine to address the belief systems of patients from foreign cultures. Some of the problem is linguistic. CLAS—Culturally and Linguistically Appropriate Services—is a set of national standards developed by the U.S. Office of Minority Health for improving communication between health care providers and patients. A medical interpreter can, on occasion, avert a tragedy. (Or cause one. When I was a medical student rotating through gynecology at Lincoln Hospital in the South Bronx, a young woman complaining of infertility was nearly given a tubal ligation because the inexperienced Spanish translator thought she was asking for sterilization.) But the potential for misunderstanding may go far beyond particular words and their definitions to a deeper level of meanings and values.

A few years ago, I took a group of medical students to Sitka, Alaska, on a field trip devoted to understanding cultural differences in medicine. Mt. Edgecumbe Hospital is a member of SEARHC— the SouthEast Alaska Regional Health Consortium—established in 1975 under the provisions of the Indian Self-Determination Act, which handed over Indian Health Service programs to tribal management. The tribal members on the SEARHC board represent the interests of eighteen communities in the region; their stated mission is to incorporate traditional Native cultural practices and values into the health care delivery system. In practice, this means a complex negotiation between twenty-first-century standards of medical treatment and old values and traditions that go back centuries.

One program that attempts to integrate Native and Western medicine is Raven's Way, a substance abuse initiative for teenagers in southeast Alaska. In traditional Tlingit culture, individuals were expected to harden the body through exercises and purify the inner self through fasting and meditation. Raven's Way uses outdoor endurance experiences on the Outward Bound model, a traditional Native diet based on local foods like berries and salmon, and group meditation to combat both drug addiction and the deeper problems of hopelessness and rage affecting the Native adolescent population. A similar program for treating substance abuse, Circle Peacemaking, is based on the "talking circle" and the tradition of the "Deer People," the peacemakers who ended clan feuds in the premodern period.

The southeast Alaska region has a tradition of observing the old customs even while beginning to adopt Western practices. One writer notes that in the 1920s, people would go to the Christian church but still practice witchcraft; they would get vaccinated for smallpox but consult the shaman "in order to play it safe." A recent example from the 1990s is the use of a "healing robe" by SEARHC patients. Sewn by a Native woman, with a totemic "Raven's Eye" figure on the back, the robe, say the people who've worn it, has emotional and spiritual powers that have led to physical healing.

Much like my patients who find comfort in organized religion and the Bible, the Native peoples of Alaska have faith in a spiritual realm separate from the mechanics of modern medicine. But unlike Jasmine Hughes and Charlotte Laszlo, who believe that good doctors have come to them from God, the Alaskan natives can feel that Western doctors fail to honor their gods. When I was in Sitka, I heard the story of a woman, eight months pregnant, who was told by the gynecologist that her baby was in a breech position and that a C-section would probably be necessary. The woman consulted a tribal healer, who took her to a steam house (*maqii,* or *banya*) to manipulate the fetus into better position for delivery. I also heard many anecdotes of people seeking traditional cures for common ailments; to take just one example, an elderly man with stomach complaints who preferred the shaman's remedies, seal oil and fish head soup, to a prescription drug for constipation.

Further back, in the 1940s and 1950s, Native people with tuberculosis were rounded up from the villages and sent into quarantine at Mt. Edgecumbe Hospital in Sitka. One hundred thirty-eight died, most of them children, and were placed in unmarked concrete caskets, which were then stacked in abandoned military bunkers. The families were never officially notified of the deaths. Historical traumas like these have understandably left the Native populations with an enduring distrust of Western medicine. All through the 1980s and 1990s, it remained a battle to get Native people to come into the hospital, even when they were critically ill and in need of admission. In recent years, the rumor revived in the villages that people had died in the hospital, and no one would agree to lie in a bed where someone had died because the dead person's spirit would haunt him. Only when the local medical director arranged for a shaman (an *ixt*) to come to the hospital and perform an exorcism of the ghosts, bed by bed, did the villagers start coming in to be admitted.

Can faith heal the sick? It's an old, and recurring, question. Among the Native peoples in Alaska, there is a tradition of mythic stories about a shaman who healed a man torn to pieces by a bear or cured a woman who was nearly burned to death. Most likely, these are fictions, but it's possible that shamans were quite effective in treating minor complaints and psychosomatic ailments, given the magical authority invested in them. The ixt were thought to be in touch with the spirit world and possessed of occult powers that could protect the village. People invested the shaman with the power to heal them; sometimes they were healed.

If belief can cure you, can unbelief (or anxiety, depression, cynicism—pick your word) make you ill? A significant literature exists, particularly in the last fifty or so years, ever since the word *stress* was appropriated from metallurgy as a medical term, supporting the notion that negative thoughts and emotions are toxic to your health. Physiological evidence points to circulating cortisol, a stress hormone, as a contributing factor in many chronic illnesses, though the question of whether cortisol (and stress in general) is a cause or effect of illness is unresolved. Nonetheless, stress is the boogeyman of our era, and belief (or positive thinking, or healthy living) is the panacea. According to a recent study, breast cancer survivors cite the following factors in preventing a recurrence: a positive attitude, 60 percent; diet, 50 percent; healthy lifestyle, 40 percent; exercise, 39 percent; stress reduction, 28 percent; prayer, 26 percent; the anticancer drug tamoxifen, 4 percent; and luck, 4 percent.[12] In my clinical experience, it's medication (and sometimes "luck") that most governs outcomes, but that's not how many patients think. Luck, though, is an interesting concept. What makes for luck? In some ways, it's a word for what we don't understand and can't control. Belief and hope, which are embedded in positive thinking, may serve some role in good outcomes in ways we don't fully grasp. But even more than outcomes, these attitudes determine how it feels to live day to day. Everyday existence depends not only on whether you're sick but also on how well you're living.

Generally, I think it's important to acknowledge our uncertainty about ultimate causes. (Even in scientific explanations of disease, a "cause" goes back only so far. If we keep asking why, there comes a point where we don't have an answer.) But along with uncertainty comes room to explore variables we don't fully understand, like the potentially positive effects of belief and optimism. From a clinical point of view, it's dangerous to posit a cause-effect relationship without any hard data, and the fact is, we're not yet in a position to mete out health credits and demerits (if, in fact, that could ever be a good idea) on the basis of people's beliefs and temperaments. But there's more to this matter of faith than simply headway against disease. Our inner landscapes make up our essence and give our days their color and texture. If hope and conviction don't necessarily affect the course of our illnesses, they unquestionably contribute to the quality of our lives.

Rose, a close friend of the family, is standing in the kitchen in one of her flamboyant getups describing the "run-in" she had with breast cancer.

"Of course you're never sure about the past tense. It's been five years, so that makes me a statistic. The good kind." She laughs her infectious laugh. "What are you going to do? You steel yourself. When I had the mastectomy, I just said, 'Now how are you going to get through this?' You can't handle it ahead of time. When you come to it, that's when you find the strength."

I've grown more comfortable asking the question, so I go ahead and ask Rose. "Does God give you strength?"

I know Rose was raised Baptist, but she says it's not really organized religion that helps her. She just has faith. She doesn't ask God for things, she gives thanks. The only time she ever asked God for anything was when she was thirty-five and her mother was very sick. "It was the one time I got on bended knee and called up on the main line and said, 'God, this is important.' When my mother died, I realized I was asking Him to do my will, not His. So now when I get up in the morning, I say, 'Thank you, God, for this day.' It's a long road, and you have to take it as it is."

Then she tells me about the "smudging."

"There's this place I go up in Wisconsin, the Red Cliff Reservation, Ojibwes and Chippewas. I went the summer after the mastectomy, and I'm wandering around—it's so beautiful there. A lake, a forest, and they have these outcroppings of rock. You'd like it there, you just put your fishing line in and, whomp, you got a fish."

I smile. She knows I'm always in the market for a new fishing hole.

"So I meet this woman who weaves baskets from white birch, she has a ninety-year-old mother who weaves too. One thing leads to another, and they take me to this hut—one of those sweat lodges. It's hot in there; they go into an altered state. So this elder of the tribe, what do you call him? Not a sachem. A shaman. He mixes tobacco and lights it, and he takes

an American eagle feather—that's very important, the eagle is sacred to them—and he waves the smoke over me. That's what they call smudging. I felt so wonderful. I felt connected to everything." She smiles. "I tell you, I wanted to be an American Indian. Of course, I was always like that. I wanted to be Jewish, I wanted to be Catholic, I wanted to be a WASP."

We laugh. Then I ask her, seriously, if she thinks the smudging ceremony healed her.

She leans against the counter and shrugs. "No, not really. But I think it was on my path of healing."

Rose's path of healing has had some memorable milestones. When she was having chemo, and her hair was starting to come out every time she combed it, she said to herself, 'Enough of this.' She filled the Jacuzzi, lit little candles, and set them around the rim. She pulled her hair back into a long braid and slipped into the tub. Then she called her husband over and said, "You get on in here with me." Colin sat behind her in the water and snipped off the braid.

I asked Rose if maybe this was a way of taking some control. Instead of all the things that were happening *to* her—surgery, chemo, radiation—here was something she could take charge of.

Rose said, "Well, you know, I never thought of that. I just thought, 'I don't want to feel bad every day watching it come out.' But that might be true. You know, find your own power."

She also told me about a ritual that helps every time she begins to feel bad. She has a chair in her bedroom that she pulls over to the window. She puts on an outfit with bright colors—oranges, yellows, whites—and sits so that the sunlight falls right on her face. "And I feel better. I said to myself a long time ago, 'I want to feel better even if I can't get better.' So I go with that. If it feels good, do it."

Rose thinks faith is an instinct, something you have inside. "It doesn't matter what you call it. Some people say God, some people call it something else. But it's there if people can just find it."

"It can't be easy," I say.

She's thoughtful. "Well, no. One thing, though, I never cried. Crying was to give in to something, to admit that something had taken me over. My brother cried, my husband cried, but not me. You just work with what you have. It's a lot of work in my head. I could have gone the other way. You say, looking back, 'Boy, that was hard; that was really hard.'" Then she shakes her head and her laugh bubbles up. "But why ask why? Just say, 'Thank you, God, for this day.'"

My patients who have the instinct for belief sometimes say they're grateful they got sick. The sickness came for a reason; it's given their lives a deeper meaning. Though I don't think of it as a gift, exactly, I too can say that my illness has given my life meaning: it's brought me closer to my patients and motivated me to help them get better. My attempt to heal others is my personal brand of faith. Maybe I can't change the course of an illness or stop death in its tracks, but I hope I can do what Rose was talking about: help someone live the best possible life, every day.

Juan Golardo has arrived on crutches that now lean against the side of his chair. He referred himself to me—his wife works for a medical supply company, and a friend in Boston said I was the one to see. Mr. G. has mineral deficiencies, which are often a sign of kidney problems. When I ask him to climb up on the examining table, he maneuvers himself carefully, sidling over with a wide, stiff-legged gait and pulling himself up with obvious effort. He seems extremely fit—muscular and trim—but his movements look like an old man's.

I consult his thick chart. He's been evaluated at a leading medical center in Florida, as well as up in New Hampshire, where he was found to have osteopenia (thinning of the bones); an MRI showed a recent rib fracture. Also, some of his laboratory results are way out of whack, particularly his phosphate, a building block of bone and teeth that's also important in cellular metabolism. He has hypophosphatemia (low serum phosphate) and hyperphosphaturia (excessive excretion of phosphate in the urine).

He's a mystery, but he's not just a "fascinoma." He's suffering. The bone pain and muscle wasting are sapping him of strength, and the absence of a clear cause is driving him crazy.

I do a regular physical exam, zooming back and forth in my chair on wheels to get my stethoscope, reflex hammer, tuning fork. Juan passes all my tests: heart and lung sounds are normal, reflexes are fine, and his peripheral vibratory sense (feet and toes) is intact. His problem is not cardiac, not neurological.

When we're facing each other across the desk, I ask him to tell me what it feels like.

"I'm a triathlete," he says. "At my peak, I was running fifty, sixty miles a week as part of my training. So when this started, I thought, 'I'm getting old, I'm overdoing it.' One doctor I saw, an orthopedist, said it was runner's knee, but it wasn't just my knee, it was everywhere, and it wasn't even related to activity. I have"—he frowns—"I can only describe them as electrical shocks. And they're out of the blue, when someone taps me on the shoulder, when I'm sitting in a chair doing nothing. It's so painful, I have to drag myself across a room."

"Sounds pretty terrible."

"It's been rough to give up running." He pauses, looks at his crutches. "Hell, running—I can't even walk. And then you know you begin to think you're crazy. Another doctor told me it was fibromyalgia, and the doctor *after that said there's no such thing as fibromyalgia. So where does that leave you? It seemed like it was my own fault."*

"How do you keep going?"

He slides a hand down the side of one crutch. "I've been a gym rat my whole life. The first year or two, I thought maybe it was a punishment for something, but now I see it more like a test." His hand goes to a small gold crucifix around his neck. "It's brought me back to God. He made me an athlete. It's His to take away."

But I don't want him to resign himself quite yet. "We need to get to the bottom of this."

"I'm doing what they told me, I take the pills. But they don't help."

Quite a lot of pills, mainly for pain: ibuprofen, naproxen, tramadol, glucosamine. I see in the chart that the endocrinologist he saw put him on low doses of calcitriol and phosphate, to help replace his mineral losses, but he's continued to excrete phosphate in his urine. No one has come up with a definitive diagnosis.

It could be his parathyroid hormone interfering with his vitamin D production, but his labs for PTH are normal. I'm hearing zebra hoofbeats: Mr. G. could have oncogenic osteomalacia, caused by a mesenchymal tumor originating in bone marrow.

"What I think we need is an MRI of your whole body. We're looking for a tumor—"

His face stiffens.

"It's a benign tumor," I say quickly. "You don't have to worry about cancer. This tumor hides all over the body, so we might have to look hard. If we can find it, though, I think it's possible we can get you back on your feet."

I don't promise him running shoes, but that, too, could happen.[13]

If my suspicions about oncogenic osteomalacia were correct, we were dealing with small disseminated tumors that secrete phosphatonins, factors affecting phosphate metabolism. Finding the tumors was important because once they were excised, Mr. G. would be returned to perfect health. So we started searching: we did a full-body MRI, then positive emission tomography (a PET scan), then computerized tomography (a CT scan). None of the imaging tests turned up the lesion—no surprise, because these tumors can hide out in connective tissue and blood, and consequently are difficult to localize. We moved on and did octreotide scintigraphy, using a radioactive isotope that binds to special receptors implicated in oncogenic osteomalacia, again to no avail. Though a newer radiographic isotope was in development, the test was not yet in wide use. That left us with venous sampling: blood collected from various points in the circulation to identify phosphatonin-secreting tumors (especially the phosphatonin fibroblast growth factor 23, or FGF23) that, so the theory goes, contribute to osteomalacia.

Here I'll take a little jaunt through some physiology. FGF23, a blood protein, is "overexpressed" in oncogenic osteomalacia. Too much FGF23 turns off phosphate reabsorption in the kidneys, with the result that phosphate is excreted in the urine. The loss of phosphate, which is necessary for bone structure and muscle energy, correlates with debility and pain. A second effect of FGF23 is to knock out vitamin D by affecting two enzymes produced in the kidneys, "downregulating" the one that's necessary to the formation of calcitriol and "upregulating" the one that deactivates vitamin D. The net result is phosphate and calcium deficiency, with attendant bone density loss and muscle pain.

All of this is very complicated, but the tests and the mechanisms tell a fascinating story about how the body hums along in balance (homeostasis) until some wily tumor comes along to interfere with normal metabolic processes, putting the whole system out of whack.

When it turned out that venous sampling, at a cost of $19,000, wasn't covered by Mr. Golardo's insurance, I continued to do what I'd been doing, slowly increasing his dosages of calcitriol, vitamin D, and phosphate to much higher levels. He began to get better, so much so that he claimed he was back to 95 percent of his old self. He'd even begun to train again—not as tough a regimen as before, but running even a few miles and lifting weights again felt wonderful. There are some worries about the future: if the tumors begin to secrete more FGF23, so that dietary supplements can't offset the losses, then we'll reinstitute the search, using the new isotope and, if that fails, pushing the insurer to cover venous sampling. But I'm content enough with the story we have: pesky tumors and metabolic screwups addressed by dietary supplements. It's a story that works. Bottom line? The patient is better.

As for Juan, he believes everything I've told him about mesenchymal tumors, FGF23, and phosphate wasting, but for him, that's not the essential story. His story is more about passing a test. God sent this to him and then sent him to me. He had a run of adversity, and now he's healed. His story is about amazing grace.

My meaning—think hard, make it better—and his meaning—keep faith and win through—come together in his happy ending. There is still something mysterious at work here. Where are the tumors? Why, really, is he better? But he *is* better.

It's dusk, and I'm standing on the porch of a rambling shingled house in Newton, Massachusetts. The windows are lit up as though it's a party, and cars are parked all the way down the street.

Mrs. Stein answers the door herself. I embrace her and say how sorry I am. She ushers me into the dining room, where the table is spread with food—exactly the food that she used to scold Mr. S. for eating: corned beef and pastrami, half-sour pickles, potato chips.

Mr. Stein was my "corned beef man." Our bargain was that he could have one sandwich a week, on Sundays. He's just died after a period on dialysis, at age eighty-four. Mrs. Stein says, "You kept him healthy for so long. He was always happy after an appointment with you." She urges me to eat. "'A good diet is one you can cheat on,'" she says, quoting him quoting me.

Mr. Stein and I had good times together. He had a long run—a longer run, I realize, than I'm likely to have. I'm pretty sure I won't make it to eighty-four the way I'm going. It's always been easier for me to be a good doctor than a good patient.

Mrs. Stein moves off to say hello to newcomers at the door. Voices drift in from the living room—they're organizing a minyan, a gathering of ten men who together recite the kaddish, the Jewish prayer of mourning, during the days after someone's death. I'm relieved to hear they've got their ten in the other room and don't need me.

I take a plate and put together a corned beef on rye in honor of Mr. Stein. Not the best food for me either, but "a good diet is one you can cheat on." As I'm eating, three older men approach me, and we identify ourselves: they're the other members of his string quartet, I'm the doctor.

"Oh, the doctor," the cellist says approvingly. "He always said you were the best. Maybe I could come see you. My blood pressure is 170 over 90."

I say, "Sure, give me a call." Meanwhile, I'm thinking, "Mr. Stein was a violinist." Something I never knew.

I finish my sandwich and move toward the entrance hall. The men in the living room are concluding the prayer, a singsong melody with soft s's and open vowels. I don't understand Hebrew. The only word I recognize is the last one: "Omeyn." Amen.

I look at the family photographs hanging on the walls of the foyer. One shows Mr. Stein as a young man, a little girl in his arms, a little boy next to him, standing in front of a white clapboard house. "That's our place on the Cape," a middle-aged woman tells me. She introduces herself: Sarah Lipton, the daughter, a lawyer with three children of her own. I say how sorry I am (why are words so inadequate?), and then I'm out on the porch buttoning up my coat.

I look up at the night sky thick with stars. Mr. Stein, a violinist. I wish I'd been able to hear him play.

5

Who Will I Be Today?

I'm meeting Cassandra Hall for the first time, after a series of screwups. I've been out of the country, and Cassandra is irritated after calling me three times and getting no response. I've arranged this meeting for the day after my return to the U.S., but we're starting off on the wrong foot.

Cassandra is blond, blue-eyed, early thirties; her nose and eyes a little red, faint circles under her eyes. She looks prickly. I've done a thorough physical exam: heart, lungs, neuro—the works. She has crackles (the technical word is rales) in her lungs, suggesting fluid in the alveoli, the tiny air sacs where gas exchange occurs, and her joints are mildly swollen. The labs the primary care provider sent over show significant protein in her urine, and she complains of shortness of breath and a persistent, "horrible" sinus problem. She's an opera singer, about to go on tour with the Handel and Haydn Society. Anything affecting her breathing and voice would be particularly problematic.

I say, "It could be lupus, but my intuition tells me it's not. Something about this doesn't fit."

Cassandra says, "So what do we do now?"

I tell her we'll get an ANCA, a blood test measuring antineutrophil cytoplasmic antibody, which will give us more information. The ANCA test is used to diagnose Wegener's granulomatosis, a life-threatening vasculitis akin to Lucy Rooney's polyarteritis nodosa, except that it affects the small vessels instead of the large arteries. I don't tell her what I'm thinking— why get ahead of ourselves?—but I do tell her to stay in town.

"I'm about to leave for Europe!"

"Wait a few days. It's important."

Cassandra folds her arms across her chest. "It better be."

The story of Cassandra's illness is unusual in several respects. First, the disease may have been a long time coming, but when it hit, it hit big, a bolt out of the blue. Coming to terms with what had happened to her, Cassandra underwent a metamorphosis. It wasn't just a matter of weaving her life back together again; because of what the disease took from her, she had to invent a new life. In the terms of this chapter, she had to "transform herself."

Cassandra's history was like that of many people who have walked around for years with an undiagnosed condition: her body was a time bomb, but she didn't hear it ticking. The way she tells it, she never experienced herself as sick. It was more like "a laundry list of things." As a junior in college, she was diagnosed with Hashimoto's, a disease affecting the thyroid gland. Then she says she forgot about it for a while. She graduated and moved to Boston. At some point, she saw a doctor about a head cold. He ordered a thyroid scan to follow up on the Hashimoto's and a chest X-ray; the scan showed a suspicious nodule, and the chest X-ray was abnormal. When she saw the surgeon about the nodule, he said, "An opera singer with thyroid cancer—a surgeon's nightmare." Amelita Galli-Curci, a famous Italian singer from the early twentieth century, permanently lost her voice after surgery for a thyroid tumor. Though Cassandra came out of the operation with her voice intact, she had several more abnormal chest X-rays.

"After that," she says, "my memory gets hazy. At some point, I had a CT scan because of the weird chest X-rays, and the radiologist asked me if I'd been around any exotic birds. Cats, yes—I had three of them—but birds, no. He insisted my lungs looked like I had psittacosis. After that, things got more and more unpleasant. I would get winded doing nothing, just sitting on the couch, and I had a cough and a runny nose all the time. The nose thing was ridiculous. I had to type holding a tissue or drippy stuff would run down my face. And when I sang, there was a noise in my ear like tinfoil crackling." A pulmonologist made her run up and down stairs with an oxygen saturation monitor on. She didn't become oxygen deprived, and she didn't get winded, so he told her, "You're not having any problems."

Cassandra says, "I thought, 'Okay, either I made this up, or it's my fault.' I decided it must be that I didn't exercise enough." But a year later, she was still having the problems the pulmonologist said she didn't have. "I was living in Charlestown near the top of Bunker Hill Street, and I'd be walking up the side street to the bus, less than a block, and have to stop before I got to the top of the hill. I was, what, thirty? It was weird. I'd say two or three words, take one or two breaths, and then I'd start hacking. It felt like there was cotton in the top of my chest. It affected my breathing but not my voice. I disguised the shortness of breath by manipulating the phrasing.

But at some point, I couldn't control the breath as I exhaled, so I couldn't finesse the ends of notes. I had no more elasticity in my lungs. Maybe someone on the street couldn't tell, but other singers knew, and anyone who was going to hire me would know."

She kept seeing the ear, nose, and throat specialist for one sinus infection after another. Then, about a year later, she visited her primary, who called the pulmonologist. Apparently, despite what he'd told Cassandra at the time, the pulmonary function tests hadn't been normal. He gave his diagnosis over the phone: sarcoidosis, an inflammatory disease that produces lumps, or granulomas, primarily in the lungs.

Cassandra says, "I went home and read up on it, but I just didn't believe him. Besides, I felt okay. It was so insidious over time, so incremental, that it had become normal. I decided against an invasive lung biopsy." Cassandra's reaction is not uncommon. In my experience, people will come into the hospital and get diagnosed with type 2 diabetes ten or even fifteen years after developing it; they present for the first time, and they already have long-term complications of the disease. Their symptoms crept up so gradually that they became a "new normal."

More months elapsed. Then, while Cassandra was getting ready to go on tour with the Handel and Haydn Society, she developed the worst sore throat she'd ever had. The primary said she had to have a urinalysis. When her urine showed 4+ protein, the doctor said, "You're seeing Julian Seifter." And that's how we met for the first time.

⁓

Our second meeting is an urgent visit. I want to start treatment right away, now that I have the results of the ANCA.

Cassandra sits opposite me, back straight, arms crossed, face wary.

I say, "It's not so good."

She shrugs. "I'm not surprised. 'Come see me first thing' is kind of a tip-off."

I tell her that the ANCA confirms what I'd suspected. What she has isn't sarcoidosis, which rarely affects the kidneys, but Wegener's granulomatosis. The disease is named for Dr. Friedrich Wegener, a physician with controversial ties to the German Nazi regime of the 1930s, and some have proposed renaming it ANCA-positive vasculitis.

"Never heard of it." She asks me to spell Wegener's; she's probably going to check it on the web as soon as she gets home. I want her to hear it from me, though. Internet descriptions tend to frighten patients with statistics and drug side effects that may not apply to them. I believe it's the job of a doctor to frame the discussion and help a person understand and weigh the data.

I explain about the inflammation of the blood vessels and the threat that poses to her vital organs, especially the kidneys. The cause is uncertain, but it's not an infection and it's not cancer. She has a 30 percent GFR—glomerular filtration rate—a measure of the effectiveness of the kidney's filtering system; this represents a significant reduction in renal function, and her lung and sinus problems most likely stem from the same inflammatory process. I stress that time is of the essence and give her the protocol, same as Lucy Rooney's. "We're going to have to treat you with steroids. Also Cytoxan. That's a chemotherapeutic agent that we hope will stop the runaway inflammation."

"Do we do it before or after?"

"Before or after what?"

"I'm going to Belgium to visit my friend and audition for work in Europe. Then I go to Scotland to meet up with Handel and Haydn. Should I wait to leave? Or do you want me to come back early?" Her arms are still folded, but it feels like she has her dukes up.

I speak slowly, distinctly. "You're not going."

I don't often lay down the law so emphatically. A few years back, I had a young patient on immunosuppressive drugs who told me that he and his wife were going camping on the Nile. I told him that, unfortunately, every organism known to man was also camping on the Nile; no way could he go there without a working immune system. The young man revised his itinerary and gave me a call: "Guess what? We're going to the Amazon!" At that point, I talked to his travel agent. Then I called him back: "Guess what? You're going on a walking tour of Scotland!"

But not even Scotland was safe enough for Cassandra, given the worsening of her disease. She started on steroids that first day, had a kidney biopsy the day after, and was on Cytoxan by the following week. (Neither the biopsy nor the Cytoxan meant cancer, as I carefully explained to Cassandra.) In talking about all this later, Cassandra says that at first she really didn't take it in. She couldn't believe that her whole life had turned upside down. Until that moment, despite her many health problems, she'd never thought of herself as ill. She says when people get married or have a baby, they think, "Wow! I'm married! I have a baby!" There's a space of "I can't believe this" while the mind catches up with the event. But people don't grant you that space when you've just been diagnosed with a life-threatening disease. Doctors want you to get it instantly; they become irritated if you're slow to understand the facts they've conveyed. But she says her brain just wouldn't cooperate in the early days.

There was one thing she did right away, the day she was diagnosed: after a rehearsal that same evening at Boston University, she asked a musician friend whether BU offered courses to people in the community. Her friend said, sure, and Cassandra immediately signed up for a course in biology. She didn't know it at the time, but she was beginning a trajectory that would carry her beyond the sickness that her mind hadn't even taken in.

The first time she understood how sick she was came, ironically, when she was experiencing the initial rush of taking steroids. "This is fantastic!" she reports thinking. "I had no idea how lousy I'd been feeling. I'd take the bus from Boston to Charlestown, thirty minutes tops, and fall asleep on the ride. I'd work, come home, eat, and fall asleep. On weekends, I'd sleep fifteen hours each day. Now, suddenly, I had all this incredible energy. By the end of two weeks, I was high as a kite, sleeping every other day, completely over the top."

Another effect of the steroids was to improve her singing, but only in bursts. She says she could suddenly hit high notes and sustain her breath uninterrupted for fifteen minutes at a time. "I felt like Glinda the Good Witch, this pure soprano coming out of me." And then, suddenly, no sound. Her vocal chords wouldn't come together; her breath just stopped. She went to the ear, nose, and throat specialist, who was expert in the effects of the medications on the airways and sinuses, and he explained that the steroid effect was only temporary; she would probably feel tired a lot of the time. But the bottom line was, the disease was going to leave her with permanent problems. Her lungs, as well as her kidneys, would experience scarring. And her voice would never be the same.

For Cassandra, the course of her illness was in many ways similar to Lucy Rooney's PAN: young woman, similar disease. The first year after diagnosis was the worst, a time of extreme, contradictory reactions. Though she didn't lose her hair on Cytoxan or become bloated and moonfaced on prednisone like many of the cancer patients in the infusion suite, she felt sick all the time. Most people didn't understand the gravity of her disease with the funny name the way they would have if it were cancer, and she felt lonely despite her friendships.

But there was one way that Cassandra was very different from Lucy Rooney. Lucy was able to have a baby and pick up the threads of her life that had been unraveled by disease. Cassandra couldn't pick up where she'd left off; for her, the cost of getting better was the loss of a long-held ambition. Even before her diagnosis, fighting for a singing career had been a struggle. Because she was always broke, she couldn't afford an audition anywhere but in Boston; she'd spent a lot of time fighting off what she thought were sinus infections and chest colds; she'd had to patch together day jobs to support herself. Now that she couldn't sing, what was she going to do?

This wasn't just a practical matter of finding a new job. Her singing was a way of living and being. She says she missed music "like you miss a person." She missed thinking musically and using the skills and language she'd worked so hard to develop. She needed to find not just a new career but a new self.

Cassandra says a key moment for her was when I described a Melitta coffee filter, one of my many analogies for kidney disease. The Melitta filter is supposed to keep back the grounds, but if holes or tears develop in the paper, then the particles flow through along with the liquid. The "particles," I explained, were the protein in her urine, which had been allowed to flow through her damaged glomeruli, the little filtration units in every nephron of the kidney.

The idea began to form in her mind that maybe she could become a doctor herself. "You just can't help teaching," she says, "and I got more and more fascinated. I think I went to med school not to stamp out disease, but to understand it."

Teaching people about disease is a big part of what I do: I instruct medical students, residents, fellows, graduate students, and there's natural spillover with my patients. Some patients, like Cassandra, are hungry for information. When I put Cassandra on methotrexate, an oral immunosuppressant to replace Cytoxan infusions, I gave her a photocopy of the clinical study that established its efficacy. When I prescribed a drug for osteoporosis or to prevent infections, I wrote out the name for her, because I knew she'd be looking it up. Scary as some of this information was, she went ahead and made herself an expert on what was wrong with her.

One day, some time in the second or third year of treatment, we were sitting in my no-frills office: desk, examining table, cabinets, and the one picture a drawing of a man that featured, for unknown reasons, the GI system. The setting didn't encourage informal conversation, but I went ahead and asked a personal question that had been much on my mind.

"You always act so peppy," I said, "but it must be hard. How do you manage all this?"

Cassandra told me later that she's very private about her feelings, but my asking made her feel less lonely. She said, "Other people are so mysterious—you never know when a word will make a big difference. When you asked me about myself, I saw that you weren't just someone who understood disease. You were someone who understood people."

This was another factor that led Cassandra to go to medical school: a wish to understand others who, like herself, had been derailed by illness. She says school itself wasn't hard, even though she was nearing forty by the time she entered. She had lots of energy, enough to run circles around her much younger classmates, and she had the capacity to take in lots of information. She says, "I just put blinders on and studied." Once in a while, she felt frustrated that she'd been near the pinnacle as a singer, and now she was starting over at the bottom. But she also loved that medicine gave her a whole new world, and a new purpose.

~

Cassandra is back for a visit. She doesn't really get followed by anyone anymore. Over the past few years, she's occasionally sent me results of her blood work from New York, where she's at medical school, but that's about it. Happily, she hasn't had a recurrence for almost five years now, and her kidney function is at 50 percent, up from 30 percent.

"Not bad," I tell her. "That's enough to be in good health."

"I feel fine, other than a little joint pain. I collect Wegener's stories, and a lot of them are gruesome. Dialysis, transplant, death. But you cured me."

"Let's hope." I'm very glad she's come through it so well. I still worry about the unpredictable nature of autoimmune diseases, but for the time being, at least, Cassandra seems pretty healthy. She'll be graduating in a month, then it's on to a residency in internal medicine in New Orleans, with plans for future training in nephrology. I ask her how medical school has been for her.

"I thought it was going to be all about intellectual mastery, but it's more than that. Maybe because I'm older, maybe because of the Wegener's, I feel I have something to tell the students, the attendings, too, about being a patient."

I smile. She still has that upright posture, that prickly air. She isn't the sort to kowtow to an attending physician.

"I know I can be a pain, but someone has to tell them."

"Tell them what?"

"That the world doesn't revolve around the doctor. That just because you explained something to a patient doesn't mean he gets it right away. That the patient still has to go home and walk the dog." She looks ready to pound the desk for emphasis.

I admire Cassandra's passion. She stands at the intersection between two worlds, and she wants doctors to be less arrogant, more responsive. She wants patients to get a fair shake.

"So," I say, "who's going to be your doctor in New Orleans?"

She shrugs. "In my opinion, the doctor should move where the patient is."

I say I'll give her a referral to someone down there, which doesn't mean she can't call me any time.

Illness changes you. Cassandra says that during the worst of her treatment, Wegener's made her self-centered, short-tempered, combative. In the end, though, she's come away with a deep empathy for people who struggle with illness. When she's in the cubicle with a patient, she's aware of the mystery of that person's life. She wants to understand, not judge. She herself has been the one on the table, in the bed, under the microscope, and she doesn't forget it.

Cassandra's transformation wasn't some miraculous rebirth; essentially, she evolved from "singer-patient" to "doctor-patient." The "patient" remains because the illness continues; the self evolves in the face of, and alongside, the sickness. Her evolution isn't the only change I've witnessed among my patients. Many others, confronting a chronic illness and an uncertain future, have changed in profound, meaningful ways. Milder variants include pursuit of a new hobby, another stab at formal education, foreign travel, new relationships, even home renovation or a personal makeover. But I'm most interested, here, in the deeper kinds of transformation: in the capacity to achieve the fluidity of identity so necessary for creative living, especially in the face of an illness that wants to box you in. At the heart of Cassandra's enterprise is reinvention—a new sense of self and purpose achieved by finding unexplored parts of the self that have been hidden by the repetitiveness of everyday life. The limitations imposed by illness, because they interrupt this repetition and challenge old arrangements, can become, paradoxically, an avenue for creative change.

Sometimes, as with Cassandra, the hidden potentials that lead to transformation reveal themselves naturally, because events invite their emergence. Sometimes, though, "transformation" is more like an ongoing series of experiments—conscious acts fueled by willful opposition to the restrictions of being sick.

Leslie Snow sits across from me, wearing an elegant dress, a silk scarf, suede boots. Her skin glows, her hair shines. In the language of medical charts, she looks "younger than her stated age" by at least a decade.

The story she's telling me is at odds with her appearance. She's had another kidney stone, another intestinal blockage, and she's worried about her urinary microalbumin test, which could be an early sign of diabetic kidney disease.

I say, "Well, here's the plus side. The fluid losses from your intestinal tract are lowering your blood pressure, which is helping your kidneys."

"You mean an ileostomy is a good thing."

I smile. "Your sense of humor's on the plus side too."

She smiles back. "I see no point in not having a sense of humor about my body. It certainly has one about me." She stands up, gathers her things. "Any instructions?"

"You're more a pro than I am about how to manage all this." She's been sick since childhood. She knows the ropes.

"Not a pro," she tells me. "More like an impostor."

Like many of my patients, Leslie has made an admirable adjustment to her illness: she's practical, resourceful, brave. But she adds to the mix a special quality all her own. She's a performance artist who brings a spirit of playfulness to the sober reality of being sick. She's never been much interested in being "herself." She'd rather invent someone new.

Leslie agreed to meet outside the office, and our conversation, stretching far beyond what an office visit would allow, gave me a more complete sense of how she manages her life, over time and day by day. It's one of the deficits of modern medicine that doctors and patients don't have more talks like this one and like the others in this book. Given the limits imposed by managed care, there's almost no place for the full narrative of an illness in the voice of the person who's sick. I've been a legal consult on many cases involving kidney failure; big boxes arrive at my door crammed with thick hospital files, but none of these files represents the human being who is (more likely than not, in a malpractice case) now dead. Though the course of a disease is thoroughly documented in the mountainous pages of hospital charts, lab reports, surgical notes, what is missing is the *experience* of the disease.

Leslie was willing to share exactly that, her private experience of a body that, as she puts it, has a wayward sense of humor. As a child Leslie had ulcerative colitis, an inflammatory disease that attacks the lining of the colon; at nineteen she underwent an ileostomy, a surgical diversion of the intestine to bypass the colon and deliver wastes into an external bag or pouch. Since then, she's had many intestinal blockages, a number of kidney stones, the onset of insulin-dependent diabetes, two kinds of early-stage breast cancer, and—more minor things—skin ailments (vaginal lichen planus and psoriasis) and narrow-angle glaucoma (an acute spike in the eye's internal pressure). Her body's sense of humor is relentless.

Leslie says one of her earliest memories is of looking out the front window of her house in Springfield, Massachusetts, wanting to go to school, but her mother said she couldn't go because she was sick. Leslie didn't understand her unending bloody diarrhea as "sick"— she had no frame of reference—but she knew her mother was anxious about it. At age six, on a night when her father had promised to bring her home cake from the wedding he was attending, she told her mother that she had a terrible stomachache, in hopes of being allowed to stay up late. Her mother grew agitated about her pains and decided Leslie should go to the hospital. In retrospect, Leslie assumes she must have been very ill that night, but she has always remembered that first hospitalization as a mistake on her part, for complaining.

At Springfield Hospital she recalls the horrible smell of the ether as she went under. The doctors had decided to do exploratory surgery, and they took out her appendix, "just in case." Leslie got her diagnosis of ulcerative colitis at that point, but the appendectomy exacerbated her abdominal problems, and she was rushed halfway across the state to Children's Hospital in Boston. There they put her on a milk diet, including milkshakes every other minute; fun at first, but awful after a while because she wasn't getting any better. They tried a new diet, and the first time Leslie saw the tray, she pointed and said, "That isn't on my diet." They were pretty impressed with a six-year-old who was so compliant, but her main aim was to get out of there. She wanted to do everything right.

This was all back in the 1950s, when much less was known about ulcerative colitis, and hospitals weren't attuned to the needs of children and parents. At one point during her stay, the doctors didn't let Leslie's father know that her bed had been moved, and he tore through the hospital, thinking she was dead. The nurses were sometimes harsh; one of them threatened to put her in a closet if she talked to her roommate at night. A psychologist was brought in, who asked her about her relationship with her older brother, and Leslie lied, saying he was the best brother in the world; he never teased her or anything. "At six I knew to protect who I was from the outside world—to construct something that would work."

After six weeks, she was released from Children's, and her doctor wrote a letter to her parents: "I'm sorry I couldn't do more to increase her chances of survival. I'm always here to talk."

Though she never saw the doctor's letter until she was an adult, Leslie began to realize how sick she was. At home she was too weak to take more than a few steps. One day, in the backyard, she realized she couldn't lift her leg to walk into the house. This terrified her.

"If you can't move, you've totally lost control." Leslie says she vowed she'd never be weak like that again. "Weakness means people can attack you. My mother used to attack me. She had a brain malignancy, seeds that kept growing in her head, and she was furious with me for adding to her stress. My father was depressed and distant, and my brother, he could be nice sometimes, but other times he'd do things like lock me out of the bathroom when I was having diarrhea. I was an outsider in my own family."

By the time she was seven, Leslie rarely went to school. She'd been an early reader, knew her multiplication tables to twelve by the time she was four, but then the learning stopped, at least in a formal sense. She felt she never learned how to write fluently, never learned much geography or history. What she did learn was how to take a proficiency test—to make it seem as though she had enough information even when she didn't. "That might have been the beginning of my career as an impostor," she says.

At school her outsider status was guaranteed by her rare attendance and by the way she looked: moonfaced, purple stripes (striae) on her legs, fuzzy hair all over her face and body—all side effects of the corticosteroids she was taking. She was emaciated. Her mother said to her, "You have to get better-looking, because you couldn't look worse." Her odd appearance was compounded by hand-me-down clothes from her much older, much shorter cousin Phyllis. The way she was perceived by her family was, "She's going to die—don't invest in her." For her sixteenth birthday, her mother gave her a stereo with the comment "I never expected you to live this long."

Leslie was also prone to storms of emotion from the steroids, but no one knew it was the prednisone. As she trembled on the verge of an outburst, her mother would taunt her, "You gonna cry now?" Leslie felt enraged by the teasing, though she didn't mind her cousin Roger's practical jokes. He once made her catch a mouse and take it outside, but that kind of thing bothered her far less than her mother's personal attacks.

In tenth grade, she had intestinal bleeding that wouldn't stop, and she went to see a Boston specialist, who told her he had no magic wand. Her mother was adamantly opposed to her having the ileostomy that would put an end to the crippling diarrhea. "No surgery, ever," she'd say. "I'm devoting my life to make sure you don't have it." After fifteen years of illness, Leslie had come to identify her whole self with her disease. She'd see the words *ulcerative colitis* and think, "That's me."

In eleventh grade, a kindly home economics teacher enrolled her in a department store competition, and they chose her to do runway modeling. Leslie figures it was because she looked like Twiggy: five foot nine, 114 pounds, with huge eyes, short hair, a scattering of freckles. Whatever the reason, it shored up her self-esteem. She developed a mantra: "It's better to look good than to feel good."

When Leslie was a sophomore in college, her mother became comatose in the hospital from the spread of the tumors and died soon after. To Leslie, this was her Get Out of Jail Free card: now she could have the surgery. Her brother warned her that no one would ever be interested in her sexually if she had the ileostomy. But Leslie's feeling was, her body was not her friend—her stomach was distended, she had stripes all over her legs and buttocks, she felt sick all the time, she couldn't go anywhere unless there was a bathroom nearby, and she was so weak she had no energy for schoolwork or outings. Still, when she took a shower the night before the operation, she stared at her abdomen and thought, "I'll never look like this again."

It was an eight-hour surgery. Her bowel was so perforated with ulcers that the surgeons had to remove it in pieces. The ileostomy "appliance" was an enormous bag; it had a holster that went around her waist with metal fittings and a vent to let out gas. The bag was so bulky that clothing was a problem. She had almost decided to wear maternity clothes and just say she was pregnant, but luckily the style in the 1960s was loose fitting, so she was able to find some outfits that would disguise the bag. "When I went back to school, my friends looked out for me. They'd guard the bathroom while I changed the appliance and wrapped up the mess in aluminum foil. Even now when I pack for the weekend, it's one-third of the suitcase for clothes and toiletries, two-thirds for medical supplies."

The year after the surgery, Leslie quickly married a man she hardly knew. She felt no one would have her; he felt she was lucky to get him. He turned out to be violent, with a psychiatric history.

He literally tried to strangle her, and after ten months, the marriage was annulled.

"Afterward, I began dating fringe guys. One of them was a Latino drug dealer, very wealthy and very polite, who wanted to marry me even though I kept saying no to sex. I never told him about the ileostomy, but I did tell some of my boyfriends. John, for example. At first he thought I was an uptight virgin because I was always avoiding physical contact. But he still wanted to sleep with me, even after I told him. Larry was an MIT guy, and he thought I was the smartest girl he'd ever met. He wanted to continue the relationship even after he saw the surgery, but his mother thought I was too big a risk. Ken, the one I married, thought I was going to tell him I was dying. He was thrilled that it was 'just' an ileostomy."

Things started to go better. There was Ken, the most important thing, and then she began to get straight As at school. After the surgery, she had much more energy, a much greater attention span. She avoided thinking about her appliance, because thinking led to obsession ("where's the bathroom, does it show, is it leaking, does it smell?"). Instead she felt freed up by the surgery, which allowed her to suppress an awareness of her body.

Leslie also began, very consciously, to build a personality. "When I caught sight of myself in a mirror, I'd think, 'Who is that person?' I'd look at other people, pick out traits I admired—calmness, wisdom, a sense of humor—and try to imitate them. I'd go through women's magazines looking at the makeup and clothing and think, 'I could be her, or her.' It never occurred to me that there was a process to becoming 'somebody.' Where educated people saw a hierarchy, a ladder to climb, I just skipped ahead; I'd show up at a job and start working. My method was to learn the lingo right away. I wanted things to sound important."

Basically, she played a role, keeping her private self private. People were impressed with her apparent command of professional language, and she portrayed herself as an attractive woman, but her real image of herself was very different: "I was the person who had ulcerative colitis, who'd had an ileostomy." When she developed diabetes and later breast cancer, she felt assaulted by the diagnoses but then shoved everything into the background. She reconstructed herself back into a whole by telling a new story about herself.

Leslie also mounted direct counterattacks to being sick; her anger has sometimes been quite useful to her as motor power to do the next thing. When she decided to become a mother, it wasn't out of any deep maternal stirrings but because, she says, "I wouldn't be denied. I wanted what everyone else had." When she couldn't get pregnant, she adopted a daughter. A few years later, she conceived a son and almost died giving birth, but she refused to be scared of life. She socialized, volunteered, took courses, changed jobs, traveled the world. Taking risks made her feel alive. As she puts it, "I like to play in the lightning."

In the two decades after the birth of her son, the specter of death was always there, looming every time she had a blockage and the dehydration persisted long enough to threaten organ failure. But she talked herself through things. "I always want a new story," she tells me. "I was tired of who I was as a teenager, I hated that story, so I kept creating new ones. Even now I talk to myself about who I am going to be today. I play around with it all the time. I have an 'under' personality that is angry, selfish, needy, and an 'over' personality that's controlled, created—the calm, caring person who is supportive of others. The facade shields me from how it really feels. I believe my facade myself, but the ugly underbelly is there too. Sometimes I'm not up to speed, something sets me off, all my vulnerabilities emerge. The needy, angry me gets in the way of my created self, the 'me' who is comfortable, attractive, successful. But then I get it all back under control.

"I'm very focused on privacy. I don't tell people what's wrong with me. Not even my children know exactly what I have. I'm great at keeping secrets, even from myself. There's a *New Yorker* cartoon I love, a man on a couch talking to his analyst: 'My feeling is, my personal life is none of my own damn business.' There are a lot of things I'd rather not think about. I prefer the stories I'm telling.

"The chief thing I carry from my childhood is a feeling of being dismissed, not cared about, not valued. I can see the humor of the falling-apart body, no pancreas, no intestine—Ken calls me Mrs. Potato Head, the woman with the screw-on parts—but I've known since I was six that bodily health is insubstantial. It all goes away no matter how young or vigorous a person is. My solution is to be the person I've created. I take pleasure in the masquerade. I know something you don't know, about life, about myself. I'm in charge."

Leslie places emphasis on the performance aspect; she's an impostor who wears costumes, recites lines, plays roles. But I think her self-description leaves out another truth: that the roles she plays are also her. It's not as though the private, needy self with the falling-apart body is the "real" one and the sophisticated competent attractive self is a fake. Both aspects belong to her. The created, chosen self has a bit of a "fuck you" in it: she is saying no to her illness, pushing back against its limits and subversions. But even if the high-gloss exterior is a protection against an inner sense of damage and neglect, it's every bit as real—as much "Leslie"—as the Leslie she's protecting. Depending on the individual, I think the best solution is sometimes a complicated one, involving play, adaptation, experiment—that "fluidity of identity" I mentioned before. We all harbor different selves inside, and being sick can enlist all of them at different times and in different ways.[14]

Both Cassandra and Leslie found ways to access submerged parts of themselves using insights gained from being ill to fight for newness and change. For myself, I have to say, once again, that my patients are better at this than I am. As I accumulated diabetes-years (which, like dog-years and light-years, are measured in different units than calendar years), my particular style of reinvention depended on the original deal I'd struck with my illness—which, as I've said elsewhere, was mostly to forget it. I couldn't use insights from my illness to transform and change because I never fully acknowledged that I was sick.

Maybe you could say I was successfully transforming myself at work, but for me, my best moments of play, experiment, and re-invention came when I traveled. Travel, for me, was my best escape from being sick, and my best opportunity to be different and express other parts of myself. I would go anywhere and try anything—which meant, in my peculiar brand of logic, that I must be just fine.

I think many of my patients share this desire for escape through adventures in the world. Cassandra was intent on traveling to Europe with the Handel and Haydn Society at the worst crisis of her illness. My young patient who reluctantly traded in a trip on the Nile for a walking tour of Scotland was likewise looking for an escape from his sickness and the limits it imposed. Leslie, too, has wanderlust—she's been on a cruise to Alaska, a tour of Europe, and a trip to Thailand, her suitcase full of ileostomy supplies.

Sometimes the drive to get away from being sick is so intense that people take considerable risks. George Richardson, another patient of mine, was just on the verge of kidney failure—his body so full of fluid that he might need dialysis any minute—when he insisted on making a trip to his second home in Florida. Not only that, but he told me he wasn't flying, he was driving, which meant that the trip down would take several days. I gave him my "You're not going" spiel, but he wasn't buying. I thought, "Well, at least it's not the Nile."

"Okay," I told him, "but you have to call me from each state you go through on the way there." In my mind, I was already compiling a list of nephrologists from all the states between Massachusetts and Florida. Three days later, after a series of phone calls from various points along the eastern seaboard, I was still waiting for one more call to say that he'd arrived. Finally, I phoned his home in Fort Lauderdale, and his wife answered. Hearing a huge racket in the background, I asked if we had a bad connection. "No," she said, "that's the rescue helicopter on the front lawn." Mr. Richardson had gone into pulmonary edema and was being medivaced to the hospital. Fortunately he recovered from that event without needing immediate dialysis, but he went on the machine as soon as he got back to Boston.

I understand Mr. Richardson's predialysis trip, as I understand the longing for much farther-flung destinations. Travel, movement, and risk are ways to stay alive, to flex muscles, to feel more whole. As the brochures tell you, It's the experience of a lifetime! It will broaden you! It will change you! It's my belief that in sickness, maybe even more than in health, we need to find the questing parts of ourselves—the desire and will to go out and experience all we can. Transformation, change, and growth depend on a store of new experiences; we are made different by the things that happen to us. Meanwhile, the burdens of chronic illness make it tempting to stay put and close the doors, retreating to a safe space where everything's known and predictable. Some people, when they become ill, hunker down; they need sameness, above all. This isn't wrong, and in fact may be quite right for certain temperaments. Not everyone is able to, or wants to, "transform."

But I still like to encourage my patients to experiment and play—to do new things and try out new roles. Sickness doesn't have to mean the end of creative living and positive transformation. In any given life, change might manifest as a major turnaround like Cassandra's, a series of playful gambits like Leslie's, or occasional action-adventure moments like Mr. Richardson's. But the impulse to imagine, play at, or experience something new is to be nurtured. "Yes, you can" is something doctors should be saying, even if it requires some negotiations about exactly what, where, and how.

I've told myself the same thing and said yes to lecture invitations all over the world: Nuremberg, Prague, Cambridge, Dublin, São Paulo, Rio, Moscow, Istanbul, Shanghai, Peking, Hong Kong, Taiwan. All those trips were ways of pushing back against my diabetes; of saying "screw you" to limitations. Each was an opportunity to change myself, if only for a time.

I'm in Mexico, on my own, my wife back at home with the kids. I've finished my lectures in Monterrey, flown to Tabasco, taken a bus to Villahermosa, and rented a car to drive into the interior and visit the Mayan ruins at Palenque. It's slow going in the jungle: dim light, rutted road; no one anywhere, just a tangle of green spreading in every direction. After what seems like forever, the ruins suddenly loom ahead of me, faintly gleaming. I get out of the car and look up at the pyramid of stones towering over me, the top obscured by thick foliage.

Slowly, carefully, feet placed sideways on the narrow steps, I climb to the summit. When I look down on the trees from the topmost ledge, I feel exhilarated. Then I have that dizzy am-I-high-or-am-I-low sensation. The way down is trickier than the way up, and by the time I reach the bottom, my heart is pounding and my vision is clouding up. I get to the car, find the candy I've brought with me, and eat it all. Somehow I make it back to my hotel in Villahermosa. By the time I get to Boston, I've polished the story for my wife: Indiana Jones and the Temple of Doom. I polish it for myself, too: I can still be on my own in the world, still brave the wilderness and make it out alive.

6

Going Fishing

Joseph Gragnano leans both elbows on the desk, lowers his head, raises his eyebrows. "So tell me, Doctor, what exactly is going on?"

This is a change of subject. So far, we've been talking about cod fishing, which Joe seems to know a lot about. I'm interested, because fishing is a hobby of mine—not one I've had much time for in my life. Joe has been explaining to me that he's good at fishing because he can think like a fish. Cod like choppy water, which is why you find them near rocks and under bridges, and they like cold temperatures, which is why you catch a lot of cod in November. I'm taking mental notes.

But now, abruptly, he's switched to his kidney. He had a transplant years ago, at age forty, and he's had some thinning of his bones, related to a long period on dialysis. We're meeting for the second time, to discuss his lab results; he just recently left his longtime kidney specialist because his insurance changed when he had to quit his job.

I always like to find out what a patient already knows. I don't want to talk down to anyone. "What did your doctor tell you the last time you saw him?"

"He said, 'You gotta take your pills.' He has me on cyclosporine, prednisone, Imuran, Procardia for blood pressure. And he's worrying about the phosphorus. I'm taking this milky stuff, a little cup every day."

"That's right, we have to correct the phosphorus. The problem is your parathyroid glands."

"Yeah, I heard about those."

I'm not sure how much Joe wants to know, but I explain anyway. "Chronic kidney disease increased your parathyroid hormone. The glands went into overdrive—it's like flipping a switch, and now it's stuck in the 'on' position. And this hormone interferes with phosphorus. The simplest thing is to take out the glands."

"You know," he says, elbows planted on the desk, "Dr. Graybar already sent me to a surgeon, and the surgeon says to me, 'Well, we're going to take out a few of the lymph nodes,' or whatever, and I say, 'Why, exactly?' And he says, 'How should I know? I'm just the surgeon.'" Joe raises his eyebrows. "I'm an auto mechanic, so I look at it a certain way. I think maybe it's like an engine, you take something out, it might not function right; like an engine doesn't work without an oil pump. So I told that surgeon no."

Good for Joe. I always think surgeons could be wrong, unless, of course, they're right. "No harm in following the bone density for a while," I tell him. "Sometimes the parathyroids readjust on their own."

Joe looks much happier about this. He pauses on his way out. "So, Doctor, I meant to ask, what's with the peeing?"

"The peeing?"

"The story is, I try and I try, and I just can't. I had that before they put me on the machine."

"Don't worry, it isn't your kidney. Sounds more like your prostate."

"Oh, right, I heard of that."

"In middle-aged men, sometimes the gland gets enlarged, like a backup, and then you have very slow urination."

He nods, then sighs. "I don't get much use out of it the other way. Sex is like those locusts that come around once every seven years."

I'm not sure what to say about the sex. "The transplant's okay, Joe," I tell him. "We'll get you a urology consult for the peeing."

Joe had a long medical history that predated his acquaintance with me. Over the course of several appointments, he filled me in on the details of his illness, from end-stage renal disease, through dialysis, and finally to transplant. Not even this latest phase has been without its problems, but Joe has a wonderful approach, a version of "just sick enough." He tends not to take in everything that doctors tell him: he mishears or misfiles information, he blocks out bad news, he goes for the bottom line—what he has to do next and what a given medical issue means for him in a practical sense. He's also developed his own theories of causation, some of them fanciful, some more realistic, but all of them useful in terms of feeling better. Joe's story is based on pragmatism, the power of positive thinking, and the idea that ignorance is sometimes bliss. He's what you might call shrewdly inattentive, an approach that's allowed him to carry on with the life he wants. Joe's story illustrates yet another strategy for transcending illness: the one I'm calling "forget yourself."

The way Joe describes it, he had "the hypertension problem" from the time he was a young man. He chalked it up to his personal troubles: he was a new immigrant from Italy trying to learn the language and fit in; he wasn't getting along with his wife, who'd married him only because she was pregnant; and he was just starting his own auto repair business.

Joe subscribes to the stress theory of disease. It was only natural that something was going to be out of whack with all these problems in his life, so he wasn't that surprised when the news came in. "I had a life insurance physical when I had my baby boy, and they told me I had too much 'albu' in my urine, whatever that is. That's when they start me on medications. The doctor, he says, 'Gotta take your pills, I can't take a crowbar and open up your mouth and shove them down.' But for me, you know, I would forget to take the pills because the blood pressure was like a drug, I could feel the energy going through me. I was working all hours, making money, getting customers from everywhere. Life was pretty good back then."

Time went by. He worked with one of his brothers, Tony, in the repair shop until the two of them had a falling-out; he hired some apprentices; he had a second child, a girl; he fought with his wife. "Stress, you know," he said. Naturally, his blood pressure was high. The doctor increased the pills, tried another brand, but the pressure stayed up, and the doctor told Joe he needed to have his kidney checked. The nephrologist turned out to be a customer of Joe's— "Jeez, I can't remember his name, a little guy with glasses, used to drive a Triumph TR3." Joe tends to know people by their cars. This nephrologist ordered an ultrasound and was the first one to tell him that he had "a serious kidney disease." He still can't tell you the name of the disease; he says they just kept calling it "the hypertension problem." Joe explained to me what the TR3 guy explained to him, which was basically a version of my Melitta filter analogy: "The kidney is like a little fine screen, and all of a sudden it's broken over here, it's broken over here, and the blood flows right through without getting clean, so you have impurity in your blood—like a car when the oil filter doesn't work."

But the doctor told him, "You're not there yet; you still have a little left." He put Joe on a no-alcohol, low-salt diet, not too much meat, a certain amount of vegetables, and pills, pills, pills. But then one day the doctor called Joe up and said he had to get a fistula—a surgically created access for needles—because he was going on dialysis any day; it was "imminent."

"We hadn't been talking about dialysis," Joe told me. "I didn't know anything about it, and I got very depressed. But in my mind, I said, 'I think they're wrong.' I go to work, come home, fall asleep on the couch, go to bed, get up at six a.m. and go to work. I still had energy. But let me put it this way: it was diminishing."

It was in the period before dialysis that Joe had an affair with a young woman. He didn't want to hurt his wife or his children; he didn't want to ruin the life of a girl twenty years younger. But: "I was in heaven. She had a little apartment, and after work I'm walking in there. She hugs me, she kisses me. You know, it's a man's dream. She's beautiful, young. She wants to marry me and have my kids. I'm not on dialysis yet, but I'm on the verge of losing my kidney, and still I feel good, I'm strong, I got a young body. She brings me life. She says, 'If you marry me, I'll give you a kidney.' Then after two, three years, she has a coworker who is falling in love with her, and I say, 'Fine, go, go.' But I did love this girl. She's leaving me, she has no choice. I stopped seeing her.

"And you know what? My kidney went. That's it. The mind and the body, boom. Something shut off."

Love, according to Joe, is antistress, but depression made the disease come into play more. "Whatever's inside of you in your body, it's there, you have it. It's like cancer cells, you have it within you, but they're waking up. You're depressed, and somehow they get energy from this, and they're waking up, and they're going to infest your body. That's what happened to me. If I kept this relationship going, it probably would not have happened for another three, four years."

But now his kidney was failing. He had the fistula created. "A few scars here and there, on my wrist, and they tie two veins together, and one of the veins came big over here." One day he nearly fainted while talking to a customer about a car problem. He went down on his knees, put his head down, his vision turned black, but then he came back to himself. The doctor said, "Ah, it's coming."

On a Saturday morning, Joe had a headache that wouldn't go away. He went into the sauna he'd built with money from the auto shop; the steam would usually clear his head. But this time, the headache wouldn't let up. He called the doctor, who said, "This is it."

"So I go over to the hospital and see this girl that the doctor told me would be waiting. She says, 'This is a dialysis machine.' I'm looking at her, I'm trembling. I wasn't feeling good, I had a headache, and I think I'm dying because I have poison in my blood. I can feel it: I have uric acid in my blood. So she says, 'We're going to dialyze you, I'm going to put the needles in you, I'm going to call your wife, okay, and tell her what time to pick you up, blah blah blah.' So she puts the needles in and starts the machine, and I see this red blood coming out of me going into the machine. I see a lot of blood running around. Where is the blood coming from? You know, it's my blood. But then, as this machine is working, all of a sudden I feel a light. My brain lightens up. I'm not feeling so sick anymore. I'm there for five hours, and I feel this refreshing in my brain, and I say, 'Oh my God, whatever it is, it's working.'"

This was the beginning of two years of dialysis, every other day.

Joe looked around to sell his business because he could die. "Reality checked in: 'Joe, sell the business.'" By now his nephrologist was no longer the TR3 guy but the doctor preceding me, who had his own dialysis suite with ten patients being dialyzed on ten machines. "I made friends there," Joe told me. "Some people died. They're not there one day, you know? But there was a guy who got a transplant, and he's fine, he's a cook. I said to myself, 'Transplant is the way I want to go.'"

It was a grueling two years. "Sometimes you'd get an infiltration in the vein, and it would hurt like crazy, but they would still have to get the needle in there. About the fistula, always a little tension there. You don't look at it, you just cover it up and watch television, and hopefully four hours was going to go by fast." Joe felt better after erythropoietin (Epogen, or EPO for short) came out, around 1988 or 1989; injections of EPO—a hormone produced by the kidney that promotes the formation of red blood cells in the bone marrow—meant he didn't have to rely on transfusions of someone else's blood. And he liked to talk to this smart, pretty girl named Stacey, a newspaper writer whose third kidney transplant had just failed. Stacey had the theory that this last kidney was no good because it had come from a gang member who'd been shot. Joe told me, "She was saying it was a bad source. I'm thinking I better be careful who my donor is."

Dialysis was always difficult, though, no matter how much he tried to get used to it. "Once I saw a guy pass out flat on his face because they took off too much fluid. The nurses give you saline, saline, saline. You get cramps sometimes on dialysis, the muscle wants to bunch up and explode, and the nurses all come and squeeze the saline thing into you, and finally it lets go. That pain is not describable."

He had some bad moments. His teenage kids never came to keep him company—Joe explains that they weren't driving yet—and his wife showed up only at the end of sessions to take him home. Sometimes he felt, "No more of this, just get it over with." "I would go down in the basement and look at my guns. I used to hunt deer, I used to hunt birds, I had a bird dog. I was actually afraid of the guns."

Joe knew people who just stopped coming in for dialysis and died in their beds. He wasn't sure how long he could keep going. He'd talked to his wife about donating a kidney to him, but she wasn't sure. She told him, "Ask your family. If they say no, we'll think about it."

Joe had been talking to his brother Rocco on the phone but never asked him for a kidney; Joe mentioned dialysis now and then, but Rocco didn't really know what it was. Then all of a sudden Rocco called him and said he was in the area, camping at Hampton Beach, and Joe should come out there and see him.

So on a sunny Saturday, Joe and his wife were walking down the beach, looking for Rocco, when they saw Rocco's camper with "Mako" written on the side, and there was Rocco himself, looking out at the ocean with his rod in the sand. Joe and Rocco hugged hello: "How you doin'?" "I'm good." "I'm good." After they got talking, Joe showed Rocco the fistula in his wrist and explained about the machine.

Rocco said, "Wow, really."

Joe explained that he was on a list for a kidney, but he didn't know when it was going to happen; it had already been a year and a half now.

Rocco said, "You need a kidney, I'll give you a kidney."

Joe said, "Yeah, right."

"No, I'm serious. I know someone at work gave a kidney to his family. I'll go home and see a doctor, see everything is okay, and then we're gonna do it."

Joe says that Rocco was always "very bold."

The two of them talked about financing. Joe agreed to pay Rocco for the time he would miss from the construction company; also, Joe's insurance would pay for both operations. Then Joe told him, "I will always recognize what you did for me." Rocco said, "No problem, don't worry about it."

Rocco got checked out by his doctor. It turned out his cholesterol was too high, and he would need to lower it before he could donate his kidney. Joe thought, "Well, that's that, he'll never do it." Then six months later, out of the blue, Rocco called and said, "I'm ready." The next time they met was in the hospital, the day before the transplant. To pass the hours, they took a walk up and down the hospital corridors. Rocco reminded Joe of the time he'd asked him for $2,000 to help with gambling debts and Joe had said no. Joe pointed out that he'd bailed Rocco out three times already—he couldn't just take it from his wife and kids and give it to Rocco every time he was in trouble. When they left to go to their separate rooms, it wasn't on such a good note, but Rocco was still giving Joe the kidney.

The next thing Joe recalled was waking up from the surgery, the nurse slapping his face and saying, "You're doing good, the kidney's working." A tube here, a tube there, a big incision with staples; pain so bad he couldn't move. Rocco came out of it fine, but now Joe had to worry about rejection. Joe's roommate in the hospital was on his second kidney.

The next morning, the doctor comes in with an entourage, Dr. This and Dr. That. They look at the roommate's chemistry, and, uh-oh, he's having a rejection. He's shaking in the bed and they put a big needle, B 52 or some kind of formula, into his catheter to kill whatever it was, and they pull the curtains with the doctors and nurses all crowded in there working on him. But the roommate stabilized. Joe didn't have to go through anything like that because his creatinine came down overnight. After he spent a couple of days walking around with the IV, they took out the staples and pulled the catheter, and he started peeing right away.

So Joe got through it well. He was also making money: he'd sold his auto repair shop, but he had a two-family house he rented out, he still held the lease on the shop, and everybody was paying rent. In this period, Rocco called up to say he needed $5,000; Rocco's girlfriend called too, urging Joe to give him the money because "he gave you life." Joe's wife objected. "No, that kidney was a gift of love. It had nothing to do with money." Joe told her, "You should have given me a kidney, you were so hesitant. My brother gave me a kidney."

Joe had a talk with his transplant doctor, who said the transplant team could help Rocco cover any medical expenses related to his kidney donation, but that was it. Joe decided to send Rocco $1,000 every month to keep him quiet.

Since the transplant, Joe has been remarkably well, although he's had a couple of near misses. After our conversation about his urination problem, he was about to go ahead with prostate surgery, but at the last minute the surgeon decided ("thank God," Joe says) that it wasn't necessary. His orthopedist recommended a double knee replacement for crippling joint pain, but Joe asked for a blood test to check for Lyme disease—his wife had just been diagnosed with it—and he, too, turned out to have Lyme. "Ticks in the backyard," Joe explained to me. "Most people would just go ahead with the knee surgery, because they think doctors are God. But doctors are human. Sometimes they're wrong. Like with a mechanic, you got a stupid little thing, and they say you need an overhaul. I say, overhaul what? So the doctor gives me a bottle of pills, and my knee problem went away."

The long course of Joe's disease is illuminating about chronicity—as the illness evolves, the strategy for managing it also evolves. What's instructive is how creative Joe's solutions have always been. His mind works on a problem in a way that is both self-protective (I don't want to know too much) and self-empowering (here's what I can do). For Joe, the glass is usually half full. His hypertension was like an energy drug; he was convinced he'd never need dialysis; dialysis, when it came, "refreshed" his brain; he made friends with other dialysis patients. And early on, he set his sights on a transplant.

Apart from putting a positive spin on what he can't fix, Joe also tends to think, like the mechanic that he is, that there's usually something you can tweak to make things run more smoothly. He interpreted his kidney failure as, in part, voluntary—he'd allowed himself to be depressed and hence vulnerable—and, consequently, he always looks for ways to keep his spirits up. He understood that Rocco was a good guy but also pretty hardheaded, so why fret over the payback for the "gift of life"? It was just part of the scheme of things and worth every penny. Joe has also had a consistently realistic assessment of doctors, using his own expertise as an auto mechanic to understand and evaluate their performance—the ones who want to do a complete overhaul, the ones who don't have a clue to what's wrong, the ones who know how to fine-tune their approach.

I haven't seen Joe in the entire last year, and he looks different: dapper, spiffy. It takes me a minute to realize it's the mustache. I compliment him on it.

"Yeah, Dr. Gill said I'd look good in a mustache. He made such a good repair I don't even need it, but I decided I like it."

Then Joe tells me the long story of his facial surgeries, explaining immunosuppression, or his version of it, as though I'm a layman and not his doctor. "You know," he tells me, "they put you on these drugs to keep the body from rejecting the kidney, and then you get these little cancers. It's the cyclosporine and the sun, because it perspires through the pores, and when the sun hits it, it generates cancer cells."

I nod. Yes, absolutely. I don't give Joe the facts—it's pretty clear he doesn't want more information from me. I'm thinking his explanation has a certain verbal logic: cyclosporine, pores.

"So I have something in my ear," he says. "It started right here. It could have been burned off, but this first doctor I saw was a butcher. He cut it out, he sewed it up, he was so proud. And there's something in my lip right here, and he cut half my lip out and sewed it back together. I looked like a dummy. And after that, there's something in my cheek over here. So I'm in for surgery, he puts an incision over here, bim bim bim, *and he cuts along the top of my nose and down and around. A hundred stitches. This doctor, he's got this blue eye. You know what? You can tell when a guy is sure what he's doing, and I don't trust this guy. I'm looking at my face, God in heaven, what happened to me?"*

I murmur something, but Joe's on a roll.

"So finally I get to Dr. Gill. He's a genius. He's got big glasses from reading so many books. He's meticulous like my grandmother when she was sewing. Dr. Gill, he fixed my nose, he fixed my lip. He said I might

have to wear a mustache. I like the mustache. At my age, it gives me character."

"You do look good," I tell him.

"Dr. Gill doesn't just cut, he burns it a little to keep things under control. He thinks like a mechanic. He's problem solving."

"Like a mechanic" is Joe's highest praise.

"You know," he says, "a doctor should be like a grandfather. My nonno used to ask me, 'How is your life?' He'd say, 'Why are you doing that?' He lived a long life, he had wisdom. A lot of doctors are too young, ta-dah ta-dah—time, money, pressure. I'm telling you."

I hope I'm not too young. I ask if he's had any other problems besides the skin cancers.

"Well, you know, I don't go as much to the Italo-American Club. I like to play bocce over there, have a drink, but I got to be careful because when I go where there are people, I could catch a cold. Anyway, a lot of people there are giving me a hard time for their own reasons."

Joe is weathering the complicated business of living with immunosuppression with his usual combination of partial knowledge, fanciful explanation, and constitutional cheerfulness. If he's getting one skin cancer after another, well, what can you do, that's his pores sweating. If he got mutilated by a butcher, well, now he's working with a genius. If he has a scar on his lip, his mustache gives him character. If public places threaten his immune system, those guys at the Italo-American Club were giving him a hard time anyway.

He keeps to his philosophy: the good offsets the bad. "I'm a positive thinker. I love adventure, I love challenges. If I were staying home watching television, thinking, 'What is going to happen next?' I'd probably be dead today. Instead I get up in the morning and say, 'What am I going to do today?' I know when the fishing season opens, the hunting season. I go out in the woods. My wife loves it up at the camp—we have a little house there by the lake. She's got her clippers on and starts trimming the bushes. We get along better now, my wife and me; in one ear and out the other. So now it's morning, a sunny day, and I look at the water—I got to go catch a fish. But first I got to do that, I got to do this, a little fixing here and there. We dig up a pine tree up on the mountain and bring it back down, we're going to plant it in our yard. We have all kinds of different trees we planted. We watch them grow. After I'm done with my chores, I get my worms, my rod. I have a little boat down at the dock. I put a big hat on to keep the sun away. And then I go fishing."

Like the other people in this book, Joe has forged a style of coping that expresses who he is. Joe's figured out how to pay the right amount of attention—which, in his case, is not too much. He's a master of the art of forgetting, something that more of us could cultivate to one degree or another. In our health-obsessed, information-crammed society, we're all supposed to be on top of it, all over it, armed to the teeth with the latest facts. But forgetting can be a capacity as well as a deficit. Deleting, blocking, or scrambling information can, on occasion, be highly adaptive. Daniel Schachter, in *The Seven Sins of Memory: How the Mind Forgets and Remembers*, points out that the mind is prone to error, even under the best of circumstances. Of his seven sins, two mechanisms of forgetting are particularly useful for anyone with a chronic illness: one is a variety of blocking (Schachter calls it repression) that involves "retrieval inhibition" of painful memories; the other is egocentric bias, the rewriting of the past to match up with positive illusions about the self.

Put another way, repression is a means of avoiding pain, and bias is a way of pursuing pleasure. The theory goes that in repression, the front part of the brain (the prefrontal cortex) sends instructions to the memory storage region (the hippocampus) to "forgeddaboutit." Meanwhile, new proteins are synthesized and neuronal connections altered every time we pull a memory out of storage, which means the memory subtly changes over time—usually in ways that make us feel better.[15]

Joe's great strength derives from exactly these maneuvers: he's willing to let bad memories slip away and happy to recall, in altered form, the "facts" that make him feel good. Neurobiology is again on his side, in the sense that stressful memories have their own natural oblivion. In *Why Zebras Don't Get Ulcers: The Acclaimed Guide to Stress, Stress-Related Diseases, and Coping*, Robert Sapolsky describes the way stress relates to memory: a little bit of arousal heightens learning, but long-term arousal eventually burns out memory. Memory burnout sounds like a bad thing, but viewed another way, a touch of amnesia can be soothing, even useful. In a chronically stressful situation, where taking action can't change things, there is little point in remembering every detail. Better to forget what's too painful and, with a little help from the sins of memory, let the picture shift into something more positive and hopeful.

Common experience suggests that we can actively help ourselves forget through meditation, soothing activity, and selective attention. At the same time, forgetting seems natural to our minds, requiring no conscious effort. According to the psychological theory of dissociation, different aspects of personality come forward under certain circumstances, while others recede. As a matter of course, we shuttle between different levels of awareness, different moods and memories, even different "selves."[16]

Let, me be clear: I'm not arguing for a permanent state of blissful oblivion. Obviously, searching out relevant information (and remembering what your doctor told you) are important means of coping with chronic illness. And there's a whole world of information readily available to those who are interested: the exploding online universe invites everyone to google their health. But first it's a good idea to determine your "information personality": are you the sort of person who thrives on facts, or does too much information overwhelm you?[17] One of the problems with internet searches for medical information is that knowing too much and remembering everything can lead to confusion and paralysis. Rusiko Bourtchouladze, a neuroscience researcher, points out that there's adaptive value in forgetting: it's only by letting go of some thoughts that we can concentrate and find perspective, "rather than rummaging indefinitely in meaningless details."[18]

In the case of cancer, the balance between attention and forgetting might be particularly difficult to achieve. The word strikes fear, even though the latest thinking is that many cancers have essentially become chronic, rather than terminal, illnesses.[19] Given the advances in treatment, which often involve a series of different tactics over time, cancer could be viewed in almost the same light as diabetes. Even so, a cancer patient may feel he is fighting for life in a more urgent way than someone with diabetes; consequently, he would do well to look into all the therapies available and be alert to new research and clinical trials.

At the same time, a certain degree of neglect or denial can be another tool for living well with cancer. A doctor with cancer faces a special challenge in this regard. Because he has so much more information than the usual patient, he's well positioned to be an active agent in the fight against the disease; but his ability to forget, and by forgetting reclaim a space to live, might be compromised by the knowledge he carries around in his head. Dr. Ron Davis, who became head of the American Medical Association in 2007 and was almost simultaneously diagnosed with pancreatic cancer, spoke of the complicated task he faced, a task made even more difficult because he was himself a physician. He educated himself on the statistics, identified errors made by his doctors, followed recommendations about diet and rest. All of this speaks to being on top of the facts. At the same time, he wanted to not think too far ahead and to cherish each day. He looked on the bright side (bald from chemotherapy, he joked that he didn't have to pack a comb or hair gel when he traveled), and he refused to resign himself to being a "goner." As he put it, "If the five-year survival rate is five percent, that's not zero." He knew, and didn't know; he remembered, and let himself forget. Or at least he tried to. He said that as a doctor, he had the advantage of understanding what was happening to him—and the disadvantage of understanding what was happening to him.[20] Still, in the time he had—he died in 2008—he lived life moment by moment, as fully as possible.

I have a patient, fifty years old, who has kidney disease related to his multiple myeloma, a cancer affecting the bone marrow. He's had chemotherapy and is doing a little better than in the past. I asked him, point-blank, how he manages to live with a bad diagnosis. He says he's a generally optimistic person, but even so, it's hard for him to forget that he's ill because he feels sick so much of the time. His body aches. In the morning, it takes him several hours to get started on the day. But he likes to sit in his easy chair; he doesn't feel sick when he's sitting there. He can listen to music, make phone calls, relax. In the easy chair, he forgets himself.

Many of my patients find a way to forget themselves—routinely, like Joe, or, if that's hard to achieve, then under special circumstances. The mind needs its protections, at least sometimes. A person needs an easy chair.

Some illnesses present worst-case scenarios that would seem to forbid one moment of forgetting, and yet, within these desperate circumstances, people still find a space to live. Decades ago, my brother-in-law—brilliant, eloquent, warm, funny—died of a rare cancer. A hematology fellow doing research at the National Institutes of Health, he came down with what looked like the flu: fevers, shaking chills, and enlarged nodes in his groin. An internist friend thought it might be mononucleosis. A surgeon friend suggested epididymitis, an inflammation of the spermatic duct. Whatever it was, it didn't go away, and finally he went to the ER. They admitted him on the infectious disease ward and biopsied the nodes; they asked him if he had cats. They were thinking it looked like toxoplasmosis, a parasitic disorder linked with exposure to cat litter.

A week or two later, looking at the odd cell type, so rare they couldn't categorize it, they decided to move him to the cancer unit. They diagnosed his illness as lymphoma and started him on chemotherapy. The regimen made him sick—hair loss, weight loss, nausea. He had a brief remission. The cancer recurred. He developed a pulmonary embolus. He underwent transfusions to replace his depleted marrow. He had a cerebral hemorrhage. And then he died. The illness, from beginning to end, lasted four months.

My brother-in-law's cancer was swiftly lethal, but, at the time, no one knew for certain when or how it would end. The family experienced his cancer as a long illness, short though it turned out to be. Minutes slowed down and expanded, as they do, in another sense, when you have a baby and enter a different kind of time. You might think that there was no space to live, but there was. We gathered around his hospital bed. When he came home, we arranged his couch in the living room. We talked, we laughed, we watched baseball. Andes mints helped with the nausea, sheepskin helped with the bedsores, Woody Allen helped with the existential dread.

During his brief remission, he cradled his newborn son and pointed out the window to the night sky, naming the constellations. He played with his three-year-old, slinging him over his back upside down and trudging across the family room asking, "Where's Austie? Has anyone seen Austie?" He filled out his Harvard College alumni questionnaire: Medical school, check. Married, check. Kids, check. Lymphoma, check. He ate a Big Mac with fries. He told a hilarious (and dirty) joke about Fokkers and Messerschmitts. He watched a dumb episode of *Hawaii Five-O*. He held hands with his wife. Even at the very end, when he realized that the bleed in his brain had robbed him of speech, he managed to express himself, smacking the IV pole across the hospital room.

The chief message of all this: you're alive until you die. Every minute counts, and relinquishing hope, playfulness, distraction, pleasure consigns you to a premature death, even when death is knocking at the door. The truth is, we're all on the same train headed for the same destination. When the diagnosis comes, forgetting it—intermittently at least—is not only understandable but sometimes quite adaptive.

The threat of death challenges the capacity of the mind to find solace. Another worst-case scenario is the "locked in" syndrome associated with amyotrophic lateral sclerosis (ALS) or massive stroke: total neurologic shutdown that robs a person of everything. How do you forget you're ill when you can't move and can't speak? One man I knew, Jules Lodish, an oncologist who developed ALS at age fifty, when asked about his long survival (he was sixty at the time), alluded to the self that escapes the prison of the body: "Much of this boils down to whether or not one can hang on to who one is . . . Quintessentially, I have found that ambulation, movement, swallowing, eating, talking, breathing, and self-care are not me. They are substantial physical losses; but they are not me."[21]

A report like this from the front lines is illuminating, because the locked-in syndrome has long been mysterious; it can look like a living death, as though the person were no longer there. But blink technology—a switch emits an infrared beam that's controlled by twitching a cheek muscle near the eye, allowing someone to key in letters on a computer board, blink by blink—has given language to those silenced by ALS, revealing how much life there is inside an apparently lifeless body. *The Diving Bell and the Butterfly*, a memoir by Jean-Dominique Bauby about his life after a massive stroke left him totally paralyzed, movingly reports his memories and his flights of imagination—the two means he has of escaping his inert body. He's able to forget himself in order to reclaim a space to live.[22]

These extreme cases point to the adaptive value of forgetting, even when the body fails completely and time is running short. In less disastrous illnesses, it's much easier to find ways to forget or, to put it more positively, to let imagination and memory roam free of the current facts. We all need to go fishing or to recline in an easy chair, to eat a Big Mac or to remember running barefoot in the grass. The self, existing within but also apart from the body, can—happily, intermittently—leave it behind. In medicine, denial often has a negative connotation, implying a flight from reality and a refusal to acknowledge important facts. In the minds of many doctors, it's the breeding ground for noncompliance and self-destructive behaviors. But denial is nearly inevitable, at least some of the time. Our minds do tend, on occasion, to disregard the facts. The trick is to harness this tendency to the good; to forget in order to create a space that transcends the hard realities of illness and allows for moments of vitality and well-being.

As I've said, denial has been my major adaptation to diabetes. But my forgetting has had phases. After years of wavering attention, it came time for me to fine-tune my approach and achieve a more useful kind of forgetting.

It's our third day in Paris, the last before our return to the States. Last week, we toured vineyards and hill towns in Provence; we're rounding out the trip with a short sojourn in Paris, where we've been racing here, there, and everywhere, seeing as much as we can in the time we have. I have a wish to be like everyone else: to be healthy and energetic, to keep pace.

This morning we're squeezing in a walk to the Luxembourg Gardens, a short distance from our hotel. We've barely gone a hundred yards when I begin to feel sweaty and dizzy. I fall behind the others, sit down on the curb; then I'm flat on the pavement, my cheek resting on asphalt. My wife is kneeling beside me, offering me sips from a bottle of Coke; a knot of people has gathered around. I hear sirens. There's an ambulance, a stretcher; hands strap me in. Up and into the dark interior. A paramedic takes an EKG while someone else hooks up a glucose drip.

Buildings race past, minutes race past; we screech to a halt. Down and out into sunlight. Up a ramp, through thick glass doors, into an examining room. The view is strange from the bed: piss green walls, low ceiling, a naked bulb over my head. My heart pounds in my chest, my breath comes in short puffs. I feel the room growing dim. Is it an embolus? An infarction? I keep my wits enough to instruct the nurse in the right way to take my pulse, counting out the beats with her: lub dub, lub dub. *I recommend* blood work and an evaluation of my blood gases. The resident, Pascale Emyard—bangs cut straight across, very calm and deliberate—raises an eyebrow. Then she tells me, "France is not a third world country."

She goes ahead with the blood gases, big needle into the radial artery just above the wrist. It should have hurt like hell, but I'm too panicked to feel pain. I look at the results with Pascale Emyard. "Very little chance it's an embolus," I suggest. Pascale, dryly, says, "No chance."

It's midnight. She decides to keep me overnight for more tests. I have the feeling she's thinking, "Crazy Harvard professor," but I don't care. I want to rule out everything dangerous.

I find out I'm at the Hôpital Laennec, a medieval château transformed, a bit imperfectly, into a medical facility. When they take me over for radiographic studies, the nurses can't fit the gurney through the narrow corridors and have to steer me across an open courtyard in the rain, a sheepskin protecting my head. We arrive at radiology (seintgraf) in the Albert Camus wing. I joke, "A good place for an existential crisis." The nurses don't laugh.

In the end, it turns out exactly as Dr. Emyard has predicted: blood sugar shifts complicated by anxiety, which caused a spike in blood pressure. She's not too impressed with my hypertension. When she gets my pressure down to 170/90, she says, "Bon. All France has that blood pressure."

Back in the States, I have a new thought. If I face my diabetes enough to fix what I can, I might be able to allow myself the thing I most desire: the luxury of forgetting. I begin to take blood sugars, before and after meals, before and after exercise. I calibrate my food and insulin accordingly. I start on antihypertensives. I take a daily aspirin. I develop a taste for tofu and bok choy. My diabetologist is delighted by my sudden compliance; I am a much better patient than I was.

Then I forgeddaboutit. And go fishing.

7

Just My Luck

Maureen Leary has just about everything wrong with her. I look at her chart and its double column of diagnostic codes: allergies, sinusitis, dry eye, migraines, syncope (fainting), urinary tract infection, eczema, dyspnea (shortness of breath), vaginitis, esophagitis, osteoporosis, arthritis, pericarditis (inflammation of the sac surrounding the heart). She's thirty years old, a flight attendant, which means travel here, there, and everywhere. How is she managing all this?

From the look of her, not well. She's semi-collapsed in her chair, and her skin, pale and lightly freckled, is almost ashen, except for a red rash that extends over the bridge of her nose to both cheeks: the butterfly rash of systemic lupus erythematosus.[23] The course of lupus is variable; some people are luckier than others in how it affects them. From the chart, Maureen doesn't seem to be having a whole lot of luck.

She hands me a sheet of lined paper on which she has written a list of ten symptoms:

1. *Numbness fingers/feet/legs*
2. *Chest pains*
3. *Pains in back*
4. *Swelling in feet, fingers, pubic area*
5. *Urine changed from yellow to dark red*
6. *Bubbles on top of feet; clear and runny liquid*
7. *Itchy pubic area*
8. *Swollen eyes, face, stomach*
9. *Period late*
10. *Pain between ribs and hip*

"You must feel pretty awful."

She makes an effort to sit erect and hold her head up. I can almost see her in a blue suit with silver wings on the lapel. "I try to be healthy," she tells me. "I take a lot of vitamins. And herbal supplements: echinacea, Saint-John's-wort, garlic, and the one for the brain, what's that called?" She laughs. "Can't remember."

"Ginkgo?"

"That's it." Her shoulders sag. "But now I have blood in my urine."

Renal problems are common in lupus. I explain that we'll do a biopsy to see exactly what's wrong with her kidneys, and then we'll organize a plan of treatment.

"I keep thinking it's my fault."

"What's your fault?"

She proceeds to tell me the story of her illness from her perspective: it began with aches and pains, skin problems, dizziness, weakness. She decided she needed exercise, vitamins, herbs. When her doctor made the diagnosis of lupus, well, that explained things, but it was still her fault.

"It's one of those autoimmune things, right?" she says. "My immune system thinks my organs are the enemy. So I began thinking, this isn't

a regular disease, this is something I'm triggering, like a war on myself. I remembered how depressed I was when I graduated college. I was living at home, I couldn't get started on my life. And then I got a cold that wouldn't go away, and all these aches and pains started, and this horrible fatigue."

"You mean you think your depression set it off?"

"I was holding things inside and fighting this endless cold, and my immune system went crazy."

"I don't think that's completely accurate."

"So tell me why I got it."

I pause. It's the question almost every patient has, though not all of them say it out loud. I stagger through an answer that sounds less like an explanation than an apology: the mechanism isn't well understood, but there may be a genetic component, an environmental component, emotional factors. But it is definitely not her fault.

She sits crumpled in the chair, her face expressionless. She doesn't believe me.

Maureen wasn't leaping to her own conclusions out of ignorance; she'd had lupus for several years before coming to me with her kidney problems, and she was up on the facts of the disease. She knew that it was mostly women who got lupus, and she knew stress played a role in flare-ups. She could recite to me the Lupus Foundation guidelines: get sleep, stick to a healthy diet, exercise when possible, take meds, stay out of the sun, try not to let emotions get out of hand.

It's one thing for the Lupus Foundation to recommend serenity, but in Maureen's mind, the advice about stress and emotion put the responsibility for flare-ups on her. Then she took it even further, to mean that her emotions had made her sick in the first place. The way Maureen saw it, she hadn't thought the right thoughts or felt the right feelings. If she had, she'd be healthy like everyone else. The simplest answer, however wrongheaded, to the "why" that haunts someone with a chronic illness is: you did this to yourself. It's a particularly tempting answer in the case of autoimmune disease. Somehow your body is getting the wrong message and turning on itself.

I'm using Maureen to introduce the theme of forgiveness, which is intimately associated with the idea of cause—or, to put it another way, blame. Our society is quick to judge people for their illnesses. In our health-obsessed, live-forever world, it's assumed that good health and long life are within everyone's control. If you're sick, it's your own fault; your lifestyle, your genes, your fault. This quickness to judge is fueled by a longing for power and safety. Even more than we want to know "why" disease happens, we want to make sure it doesn't happen to us; and the more we can blame the victim for his own ills, the safer we are.

The anxious wish to name the culprit has contributed to a puritanical, sometimes even fanatical, approach to health in our culture. I'm not promoting self-indulgence or do-nothing pessimism—there's no question that public awareness, preventive measures, and fitness recommendations are all important interventions. But I do think there's a difference between Ten Rules for Healthy Living and the Ten Commandments. Sometimes I think we've tipped too far in the direction of judgment and stigma; it's almost as though we're putting people in the stocks if they fail to meet the test of perfect self-control.

In our zealous pursuit of perfect health, we're forgetting that much medical knowledge is, unfortunately, inexact. In many cases, why someone gets sick is unknown, and how to make him better uncertain. And while we're busy censuring people for poor self-care or imagined sins of emotional excess, we're also ignoring some bedrock facts about human nature. People have psyches as well as bodies, and inside each person is a world of drives, hungers, needs, and fears, all of which may be operating in direct opposition to the Ten Rules for Healthy Living. A behavior may be implicated in an illness, but that doesn't mean a particular person will change his behavior to improve his health (or that, in fact, such a change will absolutely and necessarily lead to improvement).

I've already mentioned how stress has become associated with illness in the popular imagination: in the twenty-first century, it's our favorite cause of pathology when we don't have anything else to blame it on. Earlier times had other explanations for disease: unexpressed anger was supposed to be the cause of everything from ulcers to cancer, and sexual repression was at the root of a whole range of female complaints, from migraine to pelvic pain. Of course, stress, anger, and repression undoubtedly do contribute to the cascade of physiological and biological events that ultimately manifest as disease, but our focus on these emotional elements is double-edged. It's good to understand the contribution of feeling states like anger and fear to physiological effects like cortisol elevation or hyperventilation, but that understanding, carried to an extreme, can lead to the illusion that we could control our health if we could just manage our feelings. If stress is the boogeyman of our era, positive thinking is the panacea. But the truth is, the "cause" of most diseases is a mix of variables, not all of them well understood. We just don't know how much, or in what ways, emotion affects physical health.

In fact, what we call "diagnosis" is often dependent not on absolute scientific evidence but on a checklist of signs and symptoms.

Cancer can be diagnosed by biopsy or imaging, but many diseases can't be definitively confirmed by laboratory tests. A diagnosis of lupus, to take Maureen's case, depends on eleven criteria: malar rash (or butterfly rash, over the cheeks); discoid rash (red raised patches); photosensitivity; oral ulcers; arthritis; inflammation of the lining of the lung or heart; kidney disorder (protein or blood in the urine); blood disorder (hemolytic anemia, leukopenia, lymphopenia, or thrombocytopenia); neurologic disorder (seizures or psychosis in the absence of other causes); positive test for antinuclear antibodies (ANA); and immunologic disorder (false-positive syphilis test, among others). To be diagnosed with lupus, a person should have four or more of these symptoms, which do not need to occur at the same time. There is no single diagnostic test for the disease. You have it if you have enough signs and symptoms of inflammation to make it over the diagnostic threshold.

How, then, can Maureen think her disease is her fault? Even if exacerbations are tied to stress (as they are in multiple sclerosis and other autoimmune diseases), there's too much going on here for her to take the blame. But it's natural—inevitable, really—to develop a story of one's own experience in a way that makes private sense, even if the facts don't always bear you out. This book is full of autobiographical narratives that contain a theory of causation (or sometimes a theory of randomness). You'll remember that Joe Gragnano believed in stress as the cause of disease, while Lucy Rooney was inclined to feel that there are things you just can't control.

⁓

Several years have passed, and Maureen is back for a visit. We've reduced the protein in her urine, and her lupus is in a quieter phase. She looks a whole lot better.

She gives me a smile. "It's the Saint-John's-wort for sure."

"Give a little credit to modern medicine," I say.

Maureen shrugs. "I just have so many problems with steroids, you know?"

I nod. They are a bummer.

"You want to know what I really think?"

I nod.

"I think I moved on in my life. I got an apartment, I got a boyfriend, I took control of my life. And then all the supplements, the exercise."

I want to urge caution. Lupus is a tricky thing, and it may yet go badly for Maureen in the future. But I don't want to make her anxious either.

I say, "Good for you."

Maureen's feeling that she caused her own remission is the positive side of saying that you're in charge of your emotions and hence your fate. But as I've been saying, the negative side is equally significant. What if you can't, or don't, get well? Are you blameworthy because somehow you've failed to control your life and create a better outcome? Leslie Snow, who had an ileostomy at age nineteen and suffers from multisystem disease, thinks the notion of self-induced illness is nonsense.

"I think it's all made up. Everybody who's sick thinks they're contributing in some way, but mainly it's a wish for control. Be good, eat right, go to doctors, and it will all go away. But then you do all the right things, and guess what? You're still sick." The truth is, chance plays more of a role than is often recognized. By acknowledging chance, I don't mean to deny probable causes or undermine self-care, but to promote a kinder, less judgmental approach to the complex matter of being ill.

Of course, what looks like a cause may well be a cause, even if the statistical or laboratory evidence isn't yet in. Maureen's effort to fight off a cold might in fact have kicked her immune system into overdrive (as perhaps something similar brought on Cassandra Hall's vasculitis, when she was fighting a virus in order to perform with the Handel and Haydn Society, in chapter 5). To take another example, my brother-in-law's cancer may have been triggered by a laboratory exposure (he was the third person from that particular NIH lab to be diagnosed with a rare lymphoma), as well as by a genetic predisposition (his mother died of stomach cancer). One can speculate on what is plausible without being able to prove causation.

One not only can, one probably will. Patients do ruminate on causes—it's a basic piece of human nature to ponder why. Still, it's important to note the potential for mistakes in reasoning. *Post hoc propter hoc*—"After this, because of this"—is an error in logic that confuses temporal sequence for causation. A patient tells me, "I passed a kidney stone right after I ate a chocolate sundae," convinced it was the ice cream that caused the stone. I tell him it wasn't the sundae; it was his day-to-day diet, heavy on beer and salted peanuts, that was the likely culprit. Even so, the chances are he's going to hold on to his ice cream aversion, probably for the rest of his life.[24]

The search for causes is a search for control. Medical science attempts to identify the etiology of a disease in order to tailor treatments that will be successful in ameliorating or curing it. Patients want the safety of feeling they can influence what happens to them. But as I've stressed elsewhere, people can indulge in bad habits and risky behaviors out of that same urge to feel safe. They find an illusory sense of security in denial and acting out, or in believing that they can magically overcome the odds. They experience a thrill in saying to hell with it. They take shortcuts to pleasure through addiction, self-medicating with food, tobacco, alcohol, drugs. They think (like soldiers on a combat mission, with the bullets whizzing right and left), "It won't happen to me."

These tend to be the people whom doctors blame for their illnesses, because the causal connections are so much stronger when a disease has a significant behavioral component. These people, it appears, have chosen to be ill. But I still want to make the case for less judgment and finger-pointing. Most diseases do have some behavioral component, and most people do struggle. I see the struggle every day in my office. For example, I ask Philip Sanderson, a sixty-year-old man with hypertension and kidney disease, how he's doing with his diet. He says, "Great!" I ask him what he had for dinner last night. He says, "Wonderful scallops!" I say the scallops sound good, but the "wonderful" worries me. Breaded? Sautéed? Served in a cream sauce over noodles? People don't always know—or, in one of those dissociative blinks that the brain is so adept at, they manage to forget—that their habits are "bad." Many of the men and women I described in chapter 3, "Too Sick. Not Sick. Just Sick Enough"— the ones who wanted to believe that alcohol would hydrate their kidneys, the ones who thought they were on a low-salt diet while eating frozen pizza and SpaghettiOs—were engaged in a push-pull between denial and acknowledgment.

Patient questionnaires that probe the vulnerable areas of a person's private life—that ask about alcohol, tobacco, drugs, diet, exercise, sex—tend to be unrevealing in a climate of criticism and censure. It's like asking someone to provide ammunition for the firing squad. In my experience, the truth of patients' lives isn't always pretty; many people have a hard time coping.[25]

The reason that coping is hard is twofold. On the one hand, we often don't connect our actions with long-term consequences; that is, we don't think about the things we might be able to control. On the other hand, we simply can't know what will happen to us in the long run; that is, we realize that some things are outside our control. Optimists tend to feel confident about the future and believe they can maximize their chances for a better outcome through their own efforts. Pessimists tend to think that life is a lottery, and the world is irrational and contingent. We're all dying of something, even if we don't know what, so why bother trying to avoid the inevitable?

Preventive medicine assumes that we do have control and that we can head off certain kinds of illness if we just follow the rules. Even if that assumption were 100 percent true, people have trouble following rules. A survey commissioned by the American Diabetes Association underscores the point that there is often a disjunction between what people know they should do and what they, in fact, do. The survey reports that "more than half of Americans fear developing diabetes" and rank developing a chronic disease like diabetes as worse than losing a job, getting divorced, or falling into debt. Yet "many . . . continue the unhealthy behaviors that boost their odds of getting the blood sugar disease." The results indicated that while 70 percent of those surveyed were aware that excess weight was a risk factor for diabetes, 46 percent acknowledged being overweight; 66 percent said that avoiding doctors was risky, but 50 percent said they didn't go for medical checkups. Richard M. Bergenstal, MD, speaking for the American Diabetes Association, said many Americans "are gambling daily by ignoring risk factors for a life-altering disease like diabetes and doing nothing about it."[26]

Whether you call it gambling or denial, the minimization of personal risk comes down to the all-too-human tendency to think,

"Not me, not now." But even if we cut some slack to people struggling with things like diet and exercise, what about the drug addicts, the sexual risk takers, the alcoholics, the heavy smokers?
Shouldn't we censure them? Shouldn't we punish them?[27] Well, no.
It's not the doctor's job to sit in judgment on his patients. Besides,
such disparagement betrays a lack of understanding about the roots
of these behaviors. Genetics sometimes play a determining role: according to the disease model of alcoholism, alcoholics are to some
extent programmed to drink themselves into liver failure. Addiction
creates its own deterministic effect, stimulating the brain's reward
system beyond the reach of the decision-making and executive-
function regions of the brain.

One woman I see for kidney and blood pressure problems that
persisted after her cardiac bypass surgery told me she doesn't regret
any of the countless cigarettes she smoked in her life, though smoking is the cause of her current health problems. She leaned toward
me confidentially: "I still take the occasional puff, for old time's
sake." Patients with end-stage lung cancer have reviewed their re-
grets with me in intimate detail, telling me about the worst mistakes
of their lives at work and at home, without ever mentioning their
smoking. Maybe it was a tacit agreement between us to not name
the mistake that was killing them. And the mistake may not have
felt like a giant wrong turn or even a real decision but something
more unconscious, more in the background. They got hooked, and
afterward, at regular intervals, they argued with themselves, quit
(more than once), listened to their loved ones complain, found fellow addicts for support, and so on and so forth through many decades until, one day, the scan finally showed the spot.

I knew a lovely woman, a former ice dancer in her sixties, with a
slender frame, high cheekbones, and an enchanting smile. She'd had

a bout of nephritis, but her bigger problem was inoperable lung cancer. As we talked, she would occasionally cough discreetly into a lace handkerchief, apologizing for the interruption. I asked if she thought about it all the time. No, hardly ever. All the ice dancers smoked, she said with a shrug. That was the way it was back then.

I tell these stories to underscore that it's possible, even probable, that someone facing her own mortality can do so with a measure of self-acceptance. And I want to argue for greater acceptance of human frailty and error by doctors too. Doctors, by virtue of their training, are susceptible to fantasies of omnipotence: they know a lot, they need to know a lot, patients need them to know a lot. Playing God almost comes naturally. But it's not just doctors who fancy themselves in charge; patients, too, sometimes have dreams of omnipotence. The truth is, no health policy or medical Ten Commandments will ever entirely tame the randomness of the universe or control all the variables affecting people's health. Simply being alive means being vulnerable to time, chance, illness, death. Unfortunately, our culture is inclined to promote the illusion of invulnerability: we believe we have a right not to be ill, we think we can sidestep aging, and we avoid whenever possible the fact that each and every one of us is going to die. Why should we face facts? We have Botox! We have Viagra! We have best medical advice! If someone is sick, it's obviously his own fault.

The fact that we're all ultimately subject to the vagaries of time and chance doesn't mean we should simply throw up our hands. There's no question that we should do whatever we can to stay well. But it's an illusion to think that if we do the right things, we'll be healthy, and if we're unhealthy, it's because we didn't do the right things. Tolerance, forgiveness, and acceptance are attitudes that help us face whatever chance throws our way. It's only by acknowledging what lies beyond our control that we can fully embrace the lives we have, for the time we have them.

⌇

"Which one are you?"

The young man in the bed can barely lift his head off the pillow to ask the question. He looks worn out. Clearly, I'm at the tail end of quite a procession. I read his chart in the hallway, before I brought the team to his bedside, and he's already been seen by dermatology, hematology, rheumatology, and GI, not only at the Brigham but in his prior admission at a hospital in New Hampshire.

I can see that Michael Davis, thirty-seven, unemployed carpenter, father of a seven-month-old, and sick—very sick—is not in the mood for another consult.

"I'm the kidney guy," I tell him.

He struggles to sit up in bed; he's thin, with long hair, hollow cheeks, stubble along his jaw. "You're the one I wanted to see," he says. His voice is rough around the edges, and a faint singed odor rises off his skin: a smoker. "They told me up in New Hampshire I needed"—he stares at the ceiling, looking for the word—"hemodialysis. And I said no way, I was going down to Boston where the experts are." A shadow of a smile. "Maybe I hurt their feelings."

I tell him my name, then introduce the house staff. Michael Davis keeps his eye on me. "So, Doc, what's with my kidney?"

It isn't just his kidney. I wonder how much he understands about his situation. "I'm sure you've figured out there are a lot of things going wrong all at once."

"I'll say."

"Would you mind telling us what your symptoms are?"

He ticks them off for us, somewhat wearily—he's been asked this question a hundred times. In the last three months, he says, he's been getting sicker by the day. He's had loss of appetite, weight loss, joint pain, rashes, weakness, muscle aches, nosebleeds. He has numbness and swelling in his legs. He has stomach pain. "I've been peeing red," he adds.

I ask if he'll tell us about his life before he got sick, and he gives a quick, edited account of what's in the chart. He used to drink, some, but he's given that up. He used to smoke, but not anymore. He isn't working right now, and he worries about supporting his wife and daughter. He has another two kids by his first wife, who died of hepatitis. He's worried that maybe he has hepatitis.

I ask if I can do a physical exam, another thing he's been asked a hundred times. He sits up and lets me listen to his heart and lungs, he lies back and lets me palpate his abdomen, he dangles his legs off the bed and lets me examine the red papules—raised patches—on his calves and the red dots on his feet. I press his ankle, and the tip of my finger leaves a deep indentation: "pitting" edema. I check his reflexes, which are reduced in his lower extremities. I take his blood pressure: 190/100. The house staff hovers around.

Michael looks exhausted. "So, Doc?"

"We're going to do a biopsy to confirm what's going on with your kidney, but your blood pressure's way up and your creatinine is high, 4.1. The creatinine is a sign that your kidney isn't filtering the way it should, and your blood pressure is putting stress on the filtering mechanism, so you're putting out blood and protein in your urine."

"But what do I have?"

"We're going to find out."

"Is it serious?"

"Yes," I say, "it's serious." Among other things, he's on the brink of kidney failure. But I'm not telling him anything he doesn't know. His body has been telling him the same thing for months.

Michael leans back on the pillows. With the long hair, the skeletal frame, the look of suffering, he has a Christ-like air. "Just my luck," he murmurs.

~

"Just my luck" was Michael's shrug at the hand that fate had dealt him. But was it something as random as chance that had led him to this juncture? When I looked at the chart a second time, I saw that there was a lot Michael had left out of his personal history; specifically, IVDU—intravenous drug use—dating back ten years, and a major depression that had led to a psychiatric hospitalization and ECT, electroconvulsive therapy. A cocaine overdose that nearly killed him was most probably a suicide attempt. He'd been to Narcotics Anonymous and Alcoholics Anonymous and had apparently been clean for the last six or seven years. The smoking, which he'd claimed to have given up, was still most likely in the picture.

Out in the hall we had a miniconference, discussing diagnostic possibilities. The hematology consult had identified hemolytic anemia. The dermatologist had noted a rash on the legs consistent with systemic inflammation. The rheumatologist had diagnosed arthritis. And the GI consult had done a liver biopsy that showed evidence of hepatitis C, the thing that Michael was most worried about. A previous kidney biopsy from New Hampshire had shown membranoproliferative glomerulonephritis, inflammation of microscopic structures in the kidney caused by an abnormal immune response. The ANA, a test for lupus, and the ANCA, a test for vasculitis, had come back negative.

"So, ideas?"

"Sounds like a lot of different things," the intern suggested.

"Or one thing," the resident said.

This gave me the opportunity to launch into a discussion of two theories of causation often cited in the diagnostic literature. Of the two, the more appealing to medical sleuths is Occam's razor, which posits that the simplest explanation is the most reliable. According to this view, if we could just get to the bottom of it, we'd find a single disease at the root of Michael's myriad symptoms. Saint's triad, less of an "Aha!", proposes just the opposite: that three different findings can sometimes mean three separate disease processes. Or, as we sometimes said on rounds, quoting Hickam's dictum, "A man can have as many diseases as he damn well pleases."

I'd reached the end of my sermon. At this point, the medical student spoke up. "He injected cocaine."

Everyone swiveled around to look at her. "The liver biopsy showed hepatitis C," she pointed out. Good for her; she'd read the chart.

The intern said, "You mean you think it's the drugs? But that was, like, years ago."

The resident said, "Looks like it's come home to roost." He looked at me. "We need to cool a couple of tubes of blood."

He was thinking of cryoglobulinemia, an autoimmune disease: prolonged viral inflammation (the hepatitis C) had produced cryoglobulins, abnormal proteins in the blood that were acting as antibodies to the body's tissues and producing pathology everywhere—hence the anemia, the rash, the nephritis, the joint and muscle pain. A blood test for cryoglobulins would confirm the diagnosis. But why cool the tubes? Because the protein precipitates out only at low temperatures.

The answer, in the end, was Occam's razor. The neon signs all pointed to Michael's long-ago drug use. His fear of hepatitis was no random middle-of-the-night anxiety, as the liver biopsy had proved, and the hepatitis had triggered everything else.

The blood test returned positive for cryo, and a later kidney biopsy showed electron microscopic evidence of the protein. Michael was started on high-dose intravenous prednisone to reduce the inflammation and calcium channel blockers and clonidine to manage his hypertension. He got better. The aches went away, the rashes disappeared, the edema went down, the nosebleeds stopped; the steroids made him feel great, all around.

By the time Michael was discharged, things had improved markedly. But he wasn't much interested in causes and mechanisms. In the course of his long hospital stay, he never asked any questions about what or why. He never once mentioned to me his use of cocaine.

Michael is back in the hospital, and I've been called in to consult again. I approach the bed, put my hand on his arm. He stares up at the ceiling. He can't see me. He's had an episode of cortical blindness; his severe hypertension decreased blood flow to the visual cortex, leaving that area without oxygen.

"It's Dr. Seifter," I say.

"Hey, Doc." He gropes for my hand, gives it a shake.

"So what happened?" I ask.

"I had this splitting headache and then, boom, lights out. They say it's because I stopped the clonidine. It was making me so tired. And then the sex thing. My wife was beginning to wonder."

"We've got you on IV nitroprusside—that's another antihypertensive drug. Things should improve when we get the blood pressure down."

"I got stuff to do in New Hampshire."

I touch his arm. "It'll have to wait a little."

"How's my kidneys?"

His function is poor, but not likely to remain that way. "Let's bring your blood pressure down to earth, that's the first thing."

He doesn't look cheered up. "Man, it's been a bad year."

"I know."

Michael's bad year stretched on and on. After his initial response to corticosteroids, all his symptoms returned. He was given a trial of alpha interferon, a newer treatment that seemed promising in cryoglobulinemia, but it failed to stop the inflammation. I hadn't seen Michael for several months when I got a phone call from a colleague in St. Louis saying that a patient of mine wanted to be flown to the Brigham for treatment. Apparently, Michael had decided to go to Arizona and got so sick on the way back that he had to be taken off the train in St. Louis and hospitalized.

When I saw him at the Brigham, he was on the medical ward. He looked even thinner than last time. While in Arizona, he'd contracted a pulmonary fungal infection, coccidiomycosis, not uncommon in the desert.

I wondered where his wife and infant daughter were. Maybe the wife didn't want to travel down to Boston, but it seemed odd to me, particularly now, when his prospects of recovery were growing dim. He might never leave the hospital. Shouldn't she be here, at his side? And what about his two children from his first marriage? Why weren't they here?

He and I had always tiptoed around essential pieces of his past: the drug use, the depression. Now that his history was catching up with him, would he talk to me about his real feelings?

I began by asking him about the trip to Arizona.

"Get this, Doc. I went for the clean air." He shook his head and laughed. The pulmonary infection had come from spores in the air. "Just my luck."

"You've had a rough ride."

"Yeah." He stared out the window. "It's all heading south now."

We discussed his most recent labs and tests; he could talk the lingo like a pro by now. Creatinine, RBCs, rheumatoid factor, cryos. Then I asked him how he felt.

He shrugged.

I imagined Michael's life out of the hospital, the life he'd led when he'd had a life. He'd be wearing faded jeans, a flannel shirt, a baseball cap, work boots. No beer, no drugs, but a pack of Marlboros in his shirt pocket. He'd have a Ford pickup and a gun in the bed of the truck. Between carpentry jobs, he'd go up into the mountains to hunt deer.

I realized I was inventing this out of thin air, and what I'd come up with was the stereotype of a New Hampshire blue-collar guy: "Live Free or Die." Michael could, in fact, be full of surprises, but there was no way of knowing. He'd told me so little about himself, and he didn't seem to want to be asked.

I said I'd be by next week to see how he was doing. I knew he wasn't strong enough for dialysis, but maybe things would miraculously turn around. They didn't. Michael died before I ever got to see him again.

Was Michael to blame for his death? Was he the cause? Or was he in some sense right, that it was just his luck? The drug use establishes one starting point in the chain of events, but there are other potential beginnings. What about the depression, so severe that he'd attempted suicide? What about the relationship between the depression and the cocaine, given that drug use is sometimes an effort to self-medicate? And what about Michael's decision to go straight? Some people who cease to use drugs don't get hepatitis C or develop cryoglobulinemia.

Finally, what about the people who do well with cryoglobulinemia? Sometimes people with the disease live for a long time in relative health. Sometimes you do all the right things and the treatment works; that is, luck can be good, as well as bad. Extreme good luck—an unexplained recovery that transcends all expectation— might even be called a medical miracle.[28]

In my mind, there is enough ambiguity and uncertainty in how things go to acknowledge the notion of chance or, in Michael's words, "luck" in medical prognosis. And if Michael, who was so silent about his inner life, was invoking luck as a way to forgive himself for the past, and accept the present, I applaud him.

Sometimes a story snowballs, and it's hard, looking back, to see what caused what. Brian Casey, a neighborhood dad—forty-one years old, three kids, a job in auto parts, weekend gigs as guitarist in a rock band—saw the dentist for treatment of an abscess. He was pretty sick afterward and, figuring he needed antibiotics, went to a walk-in clinic. A "doc in the box," as Brian put it.

He got prescriptions for pain meds and some sort of penicillin-type drug, but he just got sicker: temperature of 104, shaking, chills, the works. Finally, Eve, his wife, called and told me what was happening, reminding me that Brian had a history of a heart murmur from aortic stenosis, a defect that could predispose a person to infection. I said she had to get him to the ER; I would meet them there. The intern admitted him to my medical service, where we diagnosed subacute bacterial endocarditis (inflammation of the inner lining of the heart and valves) and put him on IV antibiotics. A brief while later, I treated him for transient kidney failure, a complication of his initial infection.

Further testing showed that the tissue around his heart valve had been severely damaged by the infection, so much so that it might be impossible to put in a new one. A top-gun surgeon at the Brigham performed an exceedingly tricky valve replacement using a pig valve. None of us really expected Brian to pull through, but he did. He finally got out of the hospital after many weeks, and continued on IV antibiotics at home. It all seemed like a miracle, Eve says. He was a dead man come back to life.

At the beginning of August, a cardiologist at the Brigham, new to the hospital, urged an immediate second operation to open up the coronary vessels and clean out any remaining infection. Eve thought they should wait for the top gun to come back from Martha's Vineyard, but Brian didn't want to "wimp out." He went ahead with the procedure and, in the course of a long and complicated operation, died on the table.

Whose fault? Whose responsibility? You could look at it as tragedy (born with a defect, fated to die young). You could look at it as ironic (saved one time, but a second time, no). You could look at it as a psychological vulnerability (a tough guy, Brian was shamed into the surgery). You could look at it as bad timing (it was August, and his own cardiac surgeon was away on vacation).

Or was it just random? Brian had always talked about himself as a lucky guy, but at some point, whatever luck he had ran out. We can't know what Brian would say, but his wife, anyway, is forgiving. She says, "Who would I blame?"

Over the years, I've had my own struggles with the questions of cause, blame, chance, luck. For me, the issue of control has been a recurrent preoccupation. Diabetics need to control their blood sugars, hypertensives need to control their blood pressure, people with high cholesterol need to control their cholesterol. Whatever's out of whack, control it.

For me, this wasn't easy. As diabetes-years kept accumulating, I told myself I was doing enough to keep my house in order. At least I was testing my blood sugars and trying to adjust insulin and food accordingly. And still my disease was getting ahead of me. I began to have episodes of dizziness, with rapid pulse and sweating, almost as though I were going to pass out. I started to check my blood pressure, worrying that it was too low from the drugs I was taking, but the values suggested I was okay. I wondered if I was hypoglycemic, but again, the numbers didn't seem way out of line. Something was wrong that I couldn't get a handle on.

I decided, as Pascale Emyard had suggested in Paris, that anxiety was causing these attacks. The cure for anxiety was the boat, a Mako moored up in Newbury on the Parker River. My wife and I would go out on weekends. I'd cast for blues and stripers, and my wife would do crossword puzzles, tossing me occasional questions.

At some point, my wife hired a personal trainer for the two of us (a little to our shame; shouldn't we have been able to do it ourselves?). Jennifer turned out to be great. Spiky haired, tattooed, she'd show up on her Harley with the big handlebars and regale us with stories of wild parties, rock concerts, and Roller Derbies. It was all so fascinating, I barely noticed the exertion. Meanwhile, my wife started cooking fish and vegetables four times a week. We took walks in all weather, looking for wildlife. We spent time with our sons—family suppers, football games on TV, treks to the shore.

Things were looking up. I felt calmer, more energetic, more cheerful, more in charge, than I had in a long time. At last I was getting ahead of my disease.

~~

The alarm is buzzing. I grope for the snooze button and roll over, back to my dream, but the dream has vanished. I lie there awhile, eyes closed. I hear my wife moving around in the kitchen downstairs, and then the whir of the coffee grinder.

Okay, time to get up.

I open my eyes. What is that? There are drips of black paint sliding down the bookcase opposite the bed. I blink. I blink again. The drips don't go away.

My brain suddenly catches up to what's happening: I've had a hemorrhage in my right eye. I close the bad eye—it's been the "bad" eye for some time now—and the drips go away.

I get out of bed, fumble for my glasses. I call down to my wife, who comes running. I'm thinking, I'm blind. This is it. We rush downtown to the ophthalmologist. "We knew this could happen," Dr. Dyson says. I want to say, "It depends on what you mean by 'know,'" but I agree: yes, we knew. I open my eyes wide for the drops, then lean my forehead against his contraption and stare at the blue light moving across.

Dr. Dyson and I discuss the many laser surgeries I've had in that eye, performed to halt the slow but steady progress of diabetic retinopathy: capillaries in the eye bulge outward and then begin to leak, causing microbleeds. The laser cauterizes the affected vessels, staving off the possibility of a major bleed. Now one of those small vessels has erupted, and we're facing the full-blown hemorrhage we'd hoped to avoid.

After waiting a few weeks for my vision to clear up on its own, Dr. Dyson finally schedules a vitrectomy: he'll scoop out the jelly of my eye and inject saline to retain the shape of the eyeball. The best we can hope for is a return to my prior level of sight—not all that great, but at least I'll get light coming in from that side. I've been walking around with half the world black.

A day or two after the procedure, the bandages come off. Even though my vision is still impaired, the light has come back, restoring a measure of equilibrium. I repeat to myself what Dr. Dyson told me: any vision is better than no vision.

Dr. Dyson schedules a follow-up appointment in another month. "How's your hemoglobin A1C?" he asks casually, as we're saying good-bye. "It's been a little out of whack lately," I confess. It's true, my blood sugars have been all over the map, and I can't figure out why, exactly, what with Jennifer putting me on the treadmill and my wife serving vegetables for dinner.

He's stern. "Better get that back under control." He doesn't say it directly, but the implication is, my hyperglycemia has led to the hemorrhage.

I go through a bad period then. I am not ahead of my disease, and it's my own fault. In 1993 a major study called the Diabetes Complications and Control Trial showed that microvascular complications of diabetes—nerve, eye, and kidney disease—correlate with poor glucose control (though this fact wasn't known thirty years ago, when I first became diabetic). But it's also true that some studies show macrovascular events—heart attack and stroke—actually increase with better control because of a possible link between high insulin concentrations and atherosclerosis. Ironically, mortality increases with better control: macrovascular events are catastrophic, and hypoglycemia, a more frequent occurrence with tight control, can also be life threatening.

Was I right to be afraid of hypoglycemia? Or will that fear turn out to cause my blindness?

Then my insulin pump, a pager-sized device I wear under my shirt, breaks right before a trip I'm taking to give talks in Hawaii. It turns out *the pump hasn't been delivering insulin correctly, even though the machine has continued to show units going in at the subcutaneous site. The manufacturer says that the pump could have been failing for months, even a year.*

So what is the reason for my misfortune? I don't know for sure if the bleed was caused by decades of up-and-down sugars or by the higher glucose of the past year related to the malfunctioning insulin pump. Maybe there's some genetic factor at work, or maybe the cause is something unknown and incalculable.

Through the months that follow, I wrestle with the ambiguities and begin to accept what's happened to me. Slowly I give up the search for a single definite cause and, instead of looking back to the maybes and might-haves, take hold of the life I have. I'm ready, finally, to forgive myself. I'm ready to say "Just my luck."

8

The Growing Point

The phone is ringing. I grope for it on the end table. My glow-in-the-dark watch says seven o'clock—too early for phone calls, especially on a Sunday morning. I peer at the caller ID. Amagansett, the family summer house on Long Island.

"What's wrong?" I say into the phone.

"Hi, Uncle J." Paul's voice—my wife's sister's son.

"What's wrong?"

"It's Anne." His wife of a year, newly pregnant. "Her blood sugar's in the two hundreds, and we're worried."

I reassure him: it's okay that she's had a spike. She needs to take some insulin and check it in an hour.

Paul tells me what the doctor told them: Anne needs to keep her sugars in a narrow range, below 100. Her hemoglobin A1C should be 6. There are studies that show unstable sugars are dangerous. The pregnancy could be at risk, the fetus could be at risk. Even if the baby is born "normal," there could be hidden problems: developmental delays, cognitive issues, biologic vulnerabilities.

"Whoa, Paul." Poor kid. "Tell Anne it's okay."

By the time Paul hangs up, he's calmer.

⤳

Anne is having a "high risk" pregnancy. Because of her long-standing diabetes, she has a better-than-average chance of developing preeclampsia, a condition involving hypertension and renal problems; she could develop a serious infection; she could miscarry; the baby could be bigger than normal, necessitating a C-section. Some studies, the ones Paul was talking about, show that hyperglycemia in pregnancy means health complications for the child later on.

The standard approach to a diabetic mother is cautionary: keep your blood sugars normal, or else. The warnings are driving Anne, and by extension Paul, a little crazy. That's because, without a working pancreas, it's almost impossible to maintain a perfect blood sugar every minute of every day. I've been receiving the occasional phone call from them because I'm Dr. J., the family's personal physician, and also because, as it happens, high-risk pregnancies are one of my areas of renal expertise. Kidney disease is common in women with diabetes, lupus, and other autoimmune conditions. I consult on obstetrics all the time.

Anne's pregnancy is only one of a series of challenges she's faced in her life, beginning with her diagnosis of insulin-dependent diabetes when she was ten. For Anne, illness is no one-time event. In the course of growing into adulthood, she's had to keep finding solutions to the problems her body has posed, while remaining open to the future. Real growth, the kind we all need if we're to have meaningful lives, requires a solution that is equal parts possibility and reality. Hope and optimism—a sense of what might be—constitute the landscape of the possible. Life's limits—the hard knocks and untimely truths of lived experience—are the realm of the real. And though we like to pretend otherwise, illness and mortality are essential elements of this reality.

The task for Anne, as it is for anyone with a chronic illness, has been to walk the line between "possibility" and "reality," and let herself change and grow over time. This task is both hard and necessary; hard, because the temptation, with illness particularly, is to confine oneself to the familiar, becoming increasingly bound by habit and complacency; necessary, because only by opening oneself to what is "next" can a person truly live his life.

There are other ways to express this notion of growing through time: as a dichotomy between control and disequilibrium, or between regression and renewal. But the fundamental requirement for sustaining an authentic life as time unfolds, and as a chronic illness progresses, is to let experience change you. This idea of "growth through time," which appears in my list of maxims as the verb "grow," isn't, in fact, something you can actively do. It's a more gradual, subterranean process—a loosening of old habits, an opening up to new possibilities. When an illness takes away all your old certainties, you're almost forced into new awareness. The familiar crutches are gone, and you're left in an open state, susceptible to fresh insights and new learning. It's this open state and the subsequent reorientation that allow a person to come to what looks like "the end" and find a path forward. And this pattern—hit a roadblock, go around it—is likely to repeat many times in the course of a long illness. I'll concede that I'm talking about something similar to "transform yourself," as described in chapter 5. The difference here is that I'm more interested in those moments in an illness, often more than one, when a patient, stopped in his tracks by a difficult reality, discovers a way to grow into the future.

≥

Anne's story is particularly instructive because her disease struck in childhood; her development occurred in the context of an illness that made all the usual trials of growing up that much harder. But everyone who is ill faces something similar: the first adjustment to being sick inevitably requires revision as circumstances change.

Here's how Anne describes her first phase of coping. "I went to see the doctor because my mother was worried—I was tired all the time, thirsty, urinating. She knew the signs. The doctor immediately had me admitted to Children's Hospital. I remember learning to inject myself and then being surprised that I had to keep doing it. It was like, once, okay. But forever? That shocked me. While I was on the unit, they taught me everything about insulin and needles and glucometers and food exchanges. They told me I had to be very careful to keep my blood sugar under control or I would get the bad complications starting in ten years. In ten years, I'd be twenty-one—that was totally unreal to me. But I was scared. Maybe they wanted me to be a little scared. They'd just ended a big trial showing that tight control correlated with better health. They were really stern about what would happen if you didn't control it."

Anne's experience in the early 1990s was the diametric opposite of mine when I was diagnosed back in the late 1970s. Thirty years ago, hyperglycemia was considered the safer of the two extremes. *When* you get a diagnosis—not only how old you happen to be but also the existing state of knowledge about the disease—almost inevitably affects your attitude and coping style.

For Anne, the message was: control it or else. The other thing she remembers from her hospital stay was the girl in the next bed, older by a few years, screaming that she wouldn't take her shot. Anne didn't want to be like the screaming girl.

After a week or so in the hospital, Anne went back to her regular life, and she was a very good little girl, careful about everything. She ate the same thing for breakfast every day, tested her sugars at scheduled times, injected herself. She didn't want anyone to help her. It was her personality to want to do things on her own—she even kept her mother out of it. The one thing her mother did was inform the fifth-grade teacher. One day at school, not long after her diagnosis, Anne's blood glucose plunged to 50. She was eating candy at her desk to bring it back up when the teacher stood over her and scolded her for snacking in the middle of the school day; he took the candy and threw it in the wastebasket. Anne, too disoriented to explain herself, put her head on the desk and cried. Another kid in the class told the teacher about her low blood sugar, and the teacher apologized and retrieved the candy. He must have forgotten that she was diabetic.

It was a good thing her classmate spoke up. Anne says she didn't mind the other kids knowing about the diabetes; their knowing kept her safer. But she didn't like to inject herself in front of them, because then she felt different from the others.

Anne's first adjustment to her illness was to be a model patient— to take full responsibility for her diabetes and perfectly control her glucose. Any doctor would be delighted by such dedicated self-care. But then puberty hit: she was growing taller, her hormones were active, her body was changing. Suddenly she felt confused about her food intake, her insulin requirement. By the time she was in high school, she'd become anorexic. Not eating took care of everything at once: the less food, the less she needed insulin, and less of everything meant better control.

This accommodation worked well enough until she got to college, when, again, she was thrown off balance. "I was in my freshman year, and my roommate went away for the weekend. It was the first time I'd been alone since I got there. I woke up Saturday morning, and I was low, so I ate something. Then I took my insulin, because I was going out to breakfast with my friend. I was on two injections a day, one in the morning and one at night; I mixed fast-acting insulin with the slow-acting kind. Maybe I took two shots by mistake. I don't know for sure. When I called my friend, she wasn't ready to go yet and said she'd call me later. So I got back into bed, and I didn't wake up when she called.

"A friend wandered in—the door latch was off—and she saw I was sleeping, so she didn't bother me. She left the latch open when she went out. Then, hours later, another friend dropped in. He found me lying on the floor with a pool of blood around my head. I figure I couldn't have fallen straight out of the top bunk or I would have had bruises all over my body, so I must have started to climb out and then fallen. I don't remember anything before waking up in the hospital bed. My friend told me that when he saw me unconscious, he ran to get the residence counselor, who called an ambulance."

This event undid all Anne's previous arrangements. What if the door had been locked? What if no one had found her? Now she was afraid of not eating. She didn't feel overtly anxious, she says—she thought she was just fine—but her behavior changed. She started bingeing. She'd go to the dining hall and eat big bowls of cereal, extra bread, three kinds of dessert, sugar drinks, all in the interest of staving off hypoglycemia. In the course of her four years at college, she gained eighty pounds. At one point in her junior year, she went to see an endocrinologist, who read out her hemoglobin A1C, the laboratory blood test that indicates the level of blood sugar control. Her value was way over the target of 7, and it upset her so much that she never went back to the doctor. It wasn't the doctor, it was the number. Staring at the fact was just too much for her. Around this time, she also visited a psychotherapist, who wanted her to write down every single thing she ate. Anne fudged on the lists she handed in, and after four appointments, she quit. She says she wasn't ready to face her problems yet, though it was also a problem that the therapist was pushing facts before she'd had time to develop a relationship with him.

In the space between college and graduate school, Anne went home to live with her parents, taking office jobs and working at a day care center while she figured out what she wanted to do next. She also started seeing an endocrinologist who was a weight-loss expert. But it wasn't until she went to graduate school in psychology that Anne really addressed her eating disorder. In fact, it was only when she read the DSM (the *Diagnostic and Statistical Manual of Mental Disorders*, used by mental health professionals) that she realized that she *had* an eating disorder. She was still bingeing—unplanned bingeing—which meant she couldn't address her food intake appropriately with insulin. Wanting to figure out her problem on her own, she bought a book on diabetes and diet. But after several months, she realized she needed help and began to work with a new therapist. This therapist, unlike the previous one, never mentioned food; she asked Anne to write down not what she ate but what she felt, especially during binge episodes. By focusing on emotion, Anne was for the first time putting together her behavior and the feeling states that drove it. Anne says, for her, the therapy was a revelation.

She had always felt removed from her own feelings, unable to link her actions to her inner life. Though the therapist never spoke of what she should do in a concrete way, within a year Anne lost all the weight she'd gained in college.

Anne wrote her dissertation on eating disorders. Though she'd originally wanted to work with children, the dissertation led to a placement counseling eating-disordered patients. She's still working with that population, using her own experience to help others. One patient of hers, a forty-year-old woman with diabetes, told her about skipping insulin after eating binges in order to control her weight; basically, she was shedding sugar (and calories) in her urine. Anne told the woman that she was diabetic too and gently suggested that they look at the feelings related to overeating. Though Anne meant the disclosure as a gesture of solidarity, this woman felt that Anne was being superior and preachy. Even when Anne didn't directly reveal her illness, many of her patients found out anyway: her insulin pump would fall out of her pocket, or she'd have to excuse herself to eat something when she got low. Unlike in grade school, where having other kids know about her illness was a safety net, disclosure in the therapy setting has been complicated.

Anne met Paul in graduate school, and they married a few years later. Paul is her new safety net. Sometimes she won't wear her MedicAlert bracelet when she's out with him, because he always knows when she's low and always gets her something to eat. She hates the bracelet—a clunky ID tag that says "I'm sick"—especially now that she's acquired nice jewelry. She won't get a MedicAlert necklace because she likes her pretty necklaces.

Now Anne is pregnant, facing a new set of tensions about eating, hemoglobin A1C, self-image, and self-control. She says pregnancy is different from anything she's dealt with because she feels so responsible for the fetus. She's sharing her body with the baby and is very worried about causing harm. She's less worried about being a good mother than she is about being a good womb, at least for now. Meanwhile, her doctors tend to be reproving and anxious. The younger the doctor, the more worried, maybe from lack of experience, but also because the newer research has led to more stringent expectations in terms of glucose control. The old A1C recommendation was 7, but it's gone down to 6.5 for the general population and 6 for diabetic women who are pregnant.

Anne thinks that might be an unrealistic target, but she's trying hard. She checks her blood sugar ten times a day, she flirts with hypoglycemia often, and she tries not to overreact when her sugar's low—no panicky eating and no overshoots. Paul gets more frightened than she does when her glucometer shows a 200 reading. She knows that she sometimes hands off her feelings to Paul—he's her emotion alert as well as her medical alert. Which is why I got an early morning phone call from him, not her.

Anne's story—the good girl who became anorexic, then obese—is a story about self-knowledge and self-regulation. When Anne was starving herself and, later on, bingeing, she was wobbling to either side of the line she needed to walk. Testing the extremes may have been a way of locating the right balance. In a sense, Anne needed to bring back the little girl who followed the rules but without the anxiety and constriction of her childhood. To do that, she first needed to understand herself. The work with the second therapist, who asked her to write down her feelings when she was in the middle of a binge, allowed Anne to find her way back to herself and to a better, more balanced physical state.

I want to talk for a moment about "balance." People with chronic illness are often striving, consciously or not, for physiological equilibrium or, as physiologists like to say, homeostasis. Homeostasis is the natural condition of the healthy body: physiological mechanisms self-correct imbalances via feedback loops so that the body's machine hums along in a steady state. For example, after a meal high in salt, the normal kidney senses the salt load and preserves the appropriate sodium balance in the blood by excreting excess sodium in the urine. But the ill person lives in a body that's gone haywire. Treatments are usually aimed at restoring homeostasis: diet, exercise, medication, biotechnology, surgery are all efforts to re-create the balance that disease has destroyed. An insulin pump is, in a sense, trying to be a pancreas; a dialysis machine is trying to be a kidney. Even a transplanted kidney is trying to be a kidney. (A successful transplant requires immunosuppression, which brings its own problems. Bottom line, there's no kidney like your own kidney.)

Whatever aspects of self a person draws on—whatever knowing, transcending, forgetting he manages—the truth is, no medical intervention is as good as not needing one. Inevitably, the sick person is forced to make mental and emotional adjustments, to cede some ground to the disease even while fighting to regain control. There's always an element of making do.

Among Anne's coping skills—somewhat paradoxically, given the effort she's put into being self-aware—is a talent for forgetting. Sometimes it's helpful to forget. Though Anne is good about the restrictions of diabetes, she's not obsessive, which means she has an ability to live beyond and around what's wrong. Her in-and-out attention is a way of being herself and managing her life. But sometimes forgetting is not so good, and she needs to pinch herself into remembering.

Here's an anecdote that Anne says is pretty typical: "I was watching *The Karate Kid* on DVD with all the cousins at Amagansett. I knew I was low, but I didn't want to miss the end of the movie, and I didn't want to make a fuss about stopping it while I went and ate something, so I sat there with everyone until it was over. When I checked my sugar, it was 40. Later I realized I hadn't even followed the end of the movie, because my mind was so fuzzy."

In her efforts to minimize her illness, Anne has sometimes flirted with trouble. Now that she's pregnant, forgetting is less of an option because she'd be forgetting for two. She's entered a new phase of vigilance, not unlike her style as a ten-year-old, in order to protect the baby. You could call her pregnancy a narrative crux. For Anne, Lucy, Leslie, and other young women who are ill, being able to get pregnant and have a child are critical aims. Growth and development keep occurring, disease or no. As Benedick, the one-time bachelor turned ardent lover in Shakespeare's *Much Ado About Nothing*, puts it: "The world must be peopled!" Life has its own agenda.

But illness too has an agenda, or at least certain critical moments that shape a person's story. In my field, there are predictable crises beyond the incremental effects of progressive renal disease: the moment a patient goes on dialysis; the moment a patient gets a transplant; and the moment a transplant fails and the patient has to return to dialysis, to await another match. What aspects of self allow a person to negotiate these difficult passages? The lessons apply equally to chemotherapy, surgery, and other treatments that are uncertain and scary, yet essential.

It's not so much that people acquire a "new self" to meet a new crisis. People don't shed their old selves like a snake wriggling out of its skin. It's more that the old self, finding itself in new circumstances, adapts, changes, and grows. To repeat a familiar theme, neurobiological and psychological evidence suggests that we are made up of many selves and thus capable of many approaches. The neurobiology of learning sheds light on this inherent capacity for adaptation and change. The view that, as we age, our minds are destined to grow more rigid turns out to be inaccurate; in fact, the brain is "plastic," or malleable, and constantly alive to incoming sensations and ideas. Simply put, learning occurs when experience of various kinds (sensory, emotional, cognitive) generates electrical activity in neurons, sending strong signals down the axon (a long projection of each neural cell), and releasing neurotransmitters (chemicals such as serotonin and glutamate) that bind to receptors on neighboring neurons. Very powerful experiences result in intense, repeated stimulation of neurons, creating permanent networks that light up when we call on the information and knowledge they contain.[29]

Illness, a crisis for both body and mind, is one of those highly stimulating events that forges new structural networks in the brain. Almost inevitably, a chronically ill patient routinely gets doses of information and experience from his medical doctor, from the internet, from his illness, from life itself; it's the incoming news that, ideally, encourages new thinking and a willingness to venture forward. Very often, an "illness narrative" takes the shape of a journey into knowledge, marked by critical moments when learning occurs.[30] Some of the turning points in a story of sickness are ordinary life events: marriage, the arrival of children, career milestones, financial wins and losses, aging. The illness tends to have its own independent story line, with its own narrative cruxes: procedures, setbacks, treatments, remissions, exacerbations. Many patients, living the double narrative of their life and their illness, find their way into the next phase by simply letting themselves be changed by their experiences. They lose their balance but regain it; stopped by disease, they find a new growing point. I've often heard my patients say, "I could never face—" (fill in the blank: dialysis, chemo, amputation, colostomy, transplant, bypass). I've also seen these same people face what they said they could never face and do what they said they'd never do.

I remember Leslie Snow telling me she wasn't going to treat her newly diagnosed breast cancer; no way was she going to have a mastectomy. She was sick and tired of being "Mrs. Potato Head": no one was going to cart off any more of her body parts. I raised the point that she couldn't just jump off the moving train. The choice isn't "no breast cancer, thank you." The choice is how you withstand it—which means, in essence, choosing a treatment that's acceptable.

She decided to go back to the breast surgeon, who recommended lumpectomy, an option she could live with. The fact that she had to go through it twice, once in each breast, really made her furious; it was around then that she went to a local shooting range and learned to fire a gun. Now she has both breasts, an excellent prognosis, and a permit from the Massachusetts State Police certifying her competence with small firearms. Leslie displayed her usual playfulness in combating yet another threat and found her way to a new chapter. As she puts it, "I always want a new story."

Jules Lodish, the man I knew who had amyotrophic lateral sclerosis, developed breathing difficulties four years into the disease; he decided it was time to die and spent a tearful night preparing himself. His wife, children, and closest friends gathered around his bed, arguing in favor of the intubation that would allow him to go on, even though he was fated to a relentless decline and ultimate death. By morning, he'd changed his mind; he went to the hospital, where a breathing tube was inserted. He didn't die for another decade. Everything he ever said in the fourteen-year course of his illness suggests that, to him, his life was worth living, even though the rest of us were shaking our heads, saying "I could never—" The choice, for him, was the little bit of life he could have, or death. He chose life.

The breast lump and the respiratory crisis are critical moments when the patient has to decide on treatment or no treatment. The question of treatment comes up in geriatrics in a particularly poignant form: when someone is very old, he might wonder if there's any life left to live. When elderly patients refuse treatment, I always wonder about depression. And if it's not depression stopping them, it might be the inflexibility of mind that sometimes comes with advanced age, when it's harder to learn new things. One of the few remaining powers a sick older person has is the right to say a firm and unequivocal no. But can that person be encouraged to continue on—to remain flexible and open, and find a little bit more life ahead? Doctors themselves are sometimes less than encouraging. Advances in medicine in the last twenty years have led to successful treatments for people in their sixties, seventies, even eighties, but medicine doesn't know how to deal with ninetysomethings who are alert, engaged, and relatively well, but suffering from pain and immobility. We need a better plan of care as the average life span increases. The tendency among doctors now is to dismiss the very old patient, subtly or overtly, rather than to suggest a possible growing point into the future.

The ultimate crisis in a story of illness is the threat of death and whether it can, or should, be deferred. In my line of work, office nephrology, the major narrative crux is the moment a patient needs dialysis. Can he go forward? Or is it the end? Certainly personality influences how a person deals with such a crisis: James Michener at age eightysomething was practical and serene in the face of his late-in-life dialysis, but Bill O'Malley, the cop who liked his beer and who'd lived a much rougher, more rollicking life, couldn't accept the restraints and intrusions of a life on "the machine." In the case of transplantation, some people view the replacement organ as a miracle, like Maya Lichinsky, who was willing to live with facial cancer and the amputation of her tongue because the kidney was so valuable to her. Some, like Joseph Gragnano, appreciate the freedom from dialysis that a transplant gives. Some are terrified of immunosuppression. One woman whose kidney function is failing told me, "Don't even talk about how wonderful a transplant will be. To me, immunosuppression takes away all my defenses against the world."

A patient wrestling with feelings of helplessness and despair can't imagine a future. How can a doctor help someone accept the risk of saying yes to the unknown? How can a doctor help a patient grow?

Mr. Lee lies in the hospital bed, the sheet pulled up to his chin. His large family, all three generations, are gathered around him. They part for me as though I'm a head of state. I've already spoken to Mrs. Lee in the corridor: her husband has said no to dialysis, but the family wants him to go ahead.

Mr. Lee has an ageless face, but the chart says he's eighty-six, a retired professor of Chinese language and literature. I quickly scan his labs: creatinine off the charts, blood pressure through the roof. But aside from his kidney, the rest of him seems to be doing pretty well.

I sit down next to the bed and introduce myself. Mr. Lee and I shake hands. I ask him if he's up to talking. He nods. I thank him for giving me his time. In the back of my mind, I'm remembering an article by a Harvard psychiatrist that recommends good bedside manners as a powerful bridge to the patient. *Forget about teaching empathy to medical students; we should teach them etiquette instead.*

Mr. Lee allows his wife, children, and numerous grandchildren to leave the room. We are alone.

"How are you feeling?" I ask.

"Not well," he says. "Tired. Weak. Confused. I have a terrible head-ache."

That's the uremia, an excess of waste products in the blood; the accumulating toxins cause exhaustion and disorientation. People with end-stage renal disease can't imagine feeling better, which is why, at first, many say no to dialysis.

I explain to Mr. Lee what hemodialysis does. By pumping blood through a dialyzer—a many-layered filter that acts like a sponge—the procedure removes poisons from the blood before returning it to the body. "It's like an artificial kidney. The schedule is a little demanding; you visit the center three times a week. But people do very well with it."

"I could never live like that."

I wonder why he's so definite. Is he afraid? Is he haunted by something in his history? Or is it the depression of old age? He's emeritus, a distinguished scholar; undoubtedly, he has a wall full of honors and awards in his study at home. But maybe it all feels past tense.

"You know how much your family wants you to do this."

"But it's not their decision."

He doesn't elaborate, and I'm left with my questions. We're at an impasse. I wonder if I wouldn't feel the same if it were me—which, given my long history of diabetes, it might well be someday.

My eyes fall on a book on his bedside table. "May I?" I ask.

"Certainly."

I pick up the book, Two Views: The Collected Poems of Heng Shi. I open it: on one side of the page, a poem in Chinese, lines arrayed vertically; and on the facing page, the horizontal lines of the English translation. "Would you read one to me?"

"Certainly."

I close my eyes as he reads the English. Alternating lines describe two distinct scenes, as though two poems were weaving through each other. The sentences move back and forth between a city—streets, markets, houses—and the country—dirt path, river, birds. The city is viewed from afar, all bustle and buzz, and the country is close up: a blade of grass, a round pebble, a red wing.

I say, "It almost sounds like two voices; a man in the city and a boy in the country."

Mr. Lee smiles. "Exactly. It's between here and there, and between now and then."

He hands me the book, and I look at the Chinese side of the page: the two views flicker in the lines, like vertical blinds opening on different scenes. "You are a literature professor," I say. "You understand complexity."

He shakes his head. "Some things are simple."

"You know, you could try dialysis. See how it feels. You can always change your mind."

We look at each other, and something registers in his eyes.

In the end, Mr. Lee agreed to dialysis. Whatever vulnerabilities he had, of age, temperament, or personal history, he also had certain important things in his favor: his relative health, other than the renal issues; his large and loving family, who venerated him as an elder; and his capacity to entertain alternatives. Some people simply can't let themselves try; they are too ill, too frightened, too alone. But Mr. Lee was able to go forward and learn something new.

Perhaps because of his literary background, he had an ability to consider different perspectives and possibilities. I suspect it was this same openness of mind that helped him take the next step in treating his illness.[31]

The "next step" is something that can be encouraged rather than dismissed. It seems to me that doctors should do more than explain the facts and promote the protocol. Why not help people be more imaginative, more playful, even? Doctors can choose to accompany their patients through the trials of their illness and give them the confidence, even the permission, to keep going. The permission might be important in both subliminal and practical ways. If a doctor doesn't clearly encourage treatment, a patient may hear the message "Don't do it." Practically speaking, doctors are under pressure to justify treatments, a pressure likely to become more intense as baby boomers age and health care dollars are harder to come by. In England under the National Health Service, Mr. Lee might not even have been offered the option of dialysis because of his age. I'll leave the public health issues to the experts, but in my view, it would be a shame to deny life-saving measures to someone like Mr. Lee, healthy except for his renal failure. We are going to have many "healthy old" in the coming decades.

It's not always easy to say when a twist in the path is, in fact, "the end." Some of the choices are hard and some of the treatments grim, but the ill person, given the right encouragement, can often, despite everything, find his way to yes.

I sit across from Lyla James, a young West Indian woman, bone thin, graceful. She has serious health problems: diabetes, end-stage renal disease, AIDS.

I say, "I missed you last time."

She failed to show for her last appointment. She had the fistula done in preparation for dialysis, and in the period while the fistula was maturing, she went AWOL.

"Yes," Lyla says. She isn't much of a talker. What goes unsaid is that she couldn't face dialysis. She's dealt with AIDS and diabetes for a long time, but this newest chapter is too much for her.

"How are your blood sugars?" I'm worried about her control. She won't do as well on dialysis if her glucose stays high.

Lyla lifts her shoulders. "I don't know."

I ask if she has her glucometer, and she pulls a One Touch Ultra from her purse. The same model as mine.

"Why don't we check?"

She lifts her shoulders. "I don't understand how it works."

"I'll help you."

I show her the steps: I insert the glucose strip, set the plunger, prick her finger. A drop of blood appears. I guide her fingertip to the strip, and the machine counts down: 5, 4, 3, 2, 1. The number flashes: 183. I realize I've broken the hospital rule by doing this gloveless. It's probably the first time anyone has taken her blood without a glove in years.

Lyla rolls her eyes at the number. I smile and say, "It's not as bad as it could be." I skip a referral to the dietitian, who is culture-blind—she doesn't know anything about the typical West Indies diet, or any other national cuisine, and she hands out the same recommendations to everyone. I ask Lyla what she likes to eat—rice, beans, potato chips—and I suggest matching protein to the carbs, watching size portions, distributing calories across the day.

Toward the end of our time, I ask how she's feeling about dialysis.

Lyla lifts her shoulders. "I'll try it."

Lyla is another example of someone who "could never," and then, in the end, did. People who are sick—especially with something like AIDS, which still, despite public education, carries a lingering stigma—can feel isolated in their bodies and in need of simple contact. What I've come to realize is that the humble things count: touch that promotes an emotional connection and an awakened sense of self; casual conversation that stirs feelings of possibility and hope. Because so much of diagnosis now depends on lab tests and imaging, the physical exam, including the time-honored rituals of auscultation (listening with a stethoscope) and palpation (touching parts of the body), has become less important; but skipping it short-circuits an essential part of the healing encounter, the "laying on of hands." In Lyla's case, testing her blood sugar was a way to let her know she wasn't an untouchable but a person of worth. Talking to her about her diet was a way to help her, in some small way, imagine a future—a future that could have potato chips in it. The whole encounter allowed her to begin to come to terms with her illness, and to find a growing point.

The doctor-patient relationship, if it's trusting and warm, is crucial to good treatment. The smallest gesture can make a difference. The relationship itself can make a difference. A doctor, like a psychotherapist, can promote a playful loosening of old ways of thinking and feeling and encourage a patient to open her mind to possibilities. A doctor can help a patient grow through time.

I have some wonderful doctors myself, but because of a temperamental inability to turn myself over to another's care (and perhaps because of my doctors' kid gloves with a colleague), I've been pretty much on my own. In some ways, I've never fully faced up to the passage of time. Still, over a long period of trial and error, I think I've gained some perspective. These days, I can condense decades of living with chronic illness into a short fable: I spent years avoiding low sugars; I came to manage my glucose better; I developed retinal complications, including a hemorrhage in my right eye; I renewed my efforts at tighter control; I sought and found an inner balance.

But no moment of equilibrium is destined to last. Chronic illness is relentless, and, for me, the next complication is already under way: proliferative disease in my good eye, the left one. I have other health worries too—neuropathies that slow my walking, a Parkinsonian tremor in my hand, even a little protein in my urine (being a nephrologist hasn't protected me). But blindness is my worst fear. What will I do if I lose my sight? How will I go on living?

My wife and I are circling the lake at the college, a favorite walk of ours over the years. We've crossed the bridge, passed the mansion where the school's president lives, entered a patch of woods, and come to the topiary garden with its Edward Scissorhands trees. We stop at the parapet and look out at the water. The scene is like an out-of-focus photograph, the edges of the lake blurred, the clock tower a smudge on the horizon.

I'm remembering the day I first explained to our boys, ages two and four, what was wrong with me. I told a story about Joshua Giraffe, a character from a Raffi song. "Joshua is sick. His blood sugar gets too high when he eats his hay, and he has to take a shot of insulin to feel better. Sometimes his blood sugar goes too low, and he has to eat a candy bar to feel better." I'm still not sure how much they understood back then—they had to grow into it, the same way I did. But at the time, telling them made it really real; diabetes was a fact, incontrovertible, absolute. It seemed to me that I'd faced it once and for all. But now I see that was only the be-ginning. What's happening now feels more like the end.

"I'm going blind," I say, "but I don't care." My wife grabs my hand, squeezes it.

"The good thing is, when it happens, I won't be able to see the neigh-bors." My wife laughs and squeezes my hand tighter. I've had a low-grade irritation over the neighbor's house for years, ever since a developer built a McMansion right on the edge of our property. I've fought back with a row of arborvitae, a pergola, a fence, and still their rooftop hovers in my view. Maybe the world will go dark—in which case, I'll imagine a future that won't have my neighbor's rooftop in it.

It's fine to do without the rooftop, but what will I have left when I can't see? The rest of the way around the lake, my wife and I talk about what we'll do if the day comes. She'll read aloud to me, and we'll listen to music; we'll feel the wind together and smell the flowers; she'll cook brand-new recipes and bring me exotic foods.

There are four other senses left. "I could never—" But maybe I can.

9

Caretaking

Mrs. Valleros sits close to her husband as she explains how he's been since I saw him last. She turns her palms out and shrugs—the sleeping is not so good, but—fingers clasped—his appetite is a little better. "I watch what he's eating." She turns to her husband, touches his arm. "He sneaks salt when I'm not looking, don't you Cesare? He does! But he quotes you: 'a good diet is one you can cheat on.'" She laughs. "He loves you for that. But I think maybe the edema is not as bad as before."

Mr. Valleros sits quietly as his wife talks. He has a round face, dark hair, and dark eyes; the eyes look a little swollen despite what Mrs. V. has been saying about the edema. Cesare Valleros, president of a South American bank, conveys authority, sick though he is. He looks on with an air of satisfaction mixed with pride. His wife is beautiful, intelligent. She is keeping track of things as she should.

But despite his wife's devotion, Mr. Valleros is beginning to go downhill. Almost ten years ago, he was diagnosed with amyloidosis, a disease in which abnormal protein produced in the bone marrow accumulates in the tissues and the organs—usually the kidneys, the heart, and the GI tract. Mr. Valleros's kidney function began to decline shortly after the initial diagnosis, and he and his wife have been flying in from Buenos Aires to see me for years now. We've managed his renal disease with diet, diuretics, and medication, but the blood urea nitrogen and creatinine have increased year by year.

"We keep his feet up on pillows. I call him the Sultan." Mrs. V. smiles; her hands flutter up and settle on her husband's arm. I see how worried she is, underneath the smile.

"We're going to increase your blood pressure medication and toughen up on the diet. Do you think you can do it?" I ask Mr. Valleros.

He straightens in his chair; his wife leans toward him. He says, "We can do it."

We is the significant word here. Mr. Valleros is not sick alone. He is sick in the company and care of his wife. Many books examine the experiences of the caregiver, but it's important, I think, to look at the sick person's perspective on the one taking care of him, as well as vice versa. *Caretaker* is almost a pun. It's a synonym for caregiver, but (with a little tweak of the mind) it could just as well refer to the other person in the relationship; the one who takes, or receives, the care. That doubleness is at the heart of the partnership between the ill person and his "other," whether it's the spouse, child, parent, friend, or aide. The boundary between the two people is often porous; the need goes in both directions, and the costs, the benefits, and the ironies are often shared.

This chapter is about a final strategy of coping that occurs not within the self but between selves: the one I call "share." The word doesn't fully convey the complexity of what I mean, but it gets at one of the most difficult consequences of illness: the sudden loneliness that follows on the heels of a diagnosis. Illness separates an individual not only from the anonymous masses of "the well" but, very often, from the person closest to him, interrupting the ordinary give-and-take that existed before. Finding one's way in a couple after illness has struck is no easy task.

For every sick person and caregiver—every "couple"—very often the chief stumbling block to an authentic relationship is the problem of dependency. There are a number of different approaches to the problem, shaped by individual personality and history, but in every case the patient does better when he is willing to open himself to his partner and let another carry the burden with him. The pitfalls are many: the caregiver can become too powerful or controlling, or too enslaved and overwhelmed; the sick person can become a demanding invalid or a captive of a kind. In short, the patient-caregiver relationship is like every relationship: will it be a power struggle or a fruitful collaboration? The benefits of a good partnership between the caretaker and the caregiver are profound: working together, a good pair can minimize the intrusiveness of illness and sustain a sense of normalcy, continuity, perspective. They can allow themselves the sort of back-and-forth—sometimes harmonious and sometimes contentious—that promotes liveliness and growth.

For Mr. and Mrs. Valleros, the arrangement looked easy, even delightful. Mrs. V.—Miranda—was the expressive one, the interpreter and translator; she was the manager, too, who handled the diet, the meds, the day-to-day care. She looked to be in charge, but Mr. V. radiated quiet power. He was a captain of finance, used to delegating authority, and he seemed completely comfortable turning over the daily business of his sickness to his wife. She was the senior vice president of everything, but there was no mistaking who was president. Even his silences were powerful: he was taking it all in, assessing performance and probabilities.

There was also, for the Valleroses, the matter of money. They had a lot of it, which provided a buffer zone of comfort. Their apartment in Boston had a stunning view of the harbor and the river; there were fresh flowers on the sideboard, fresh fruit on the table, marble floors and Oriental rugs, plush furniture and handsome art. They invited my wife and me for a visit, and their whole family, five daughters and two sons, was there. Several were married, with young children. Also, the youngest daughter had just become engaged, and there were plans under way for a big wedding in Buenos Aires. Cesare's sickness was the reason they had gathered in Boston, but the subject was delicately sidestepped. The children were running down the marble halls, the menus for the wedding had to be decided. They were in the thick of life, even as his health ebbed.

Possibly I've idealized this couple, but in all the years of our acquaintance, I never saw a whiff of blame or resentment pass between them. They were gracious, kind people. They even had a mass said for me at the cathedral in Buenos Aires—not that I completely understood what that meant in a religious sense, but I felt honored by the gesture. When I visited their Boston apartment a second time, late in the illness, Miranda cried with me when Cesare was out of the room. When he died, I met with her in my office, and she showed me pictures from her daughter's wedding and snapshots of the grandchildren.

The Valleroses' wealth did help: they could afford to come to the Brigham for his care, and they could support a second home and a staff of servants and aides. But in the end, money doesn't change the course of a disease. We are all, as King Lear says, "poor, bare, fork'd animals" once you take away our finery. What distinguishes the Valleroses in my mind is not their wealth but their relationship. It seems to me that they drew on their natural strengths—her vivacity and energy, his skill at analyzing and managing, and their mutual devotion—to make the long course of his illness as tolerable, and as meaningful, as possible.

The collaboration of the Valleroses seemed effortless and natural, but many other pairs I've encountered have found collaborating hard work. A marriage requires room for two, and illness tends to constrict the space. How can a couple thrive when it's so easy to let illness close things down in ways that stunt growth and liveliness? How can the necessary collisions between two different people be fruitful rather than bruising? One way is to put the illness in its place.

Leslie Snow, my longtime patient with the ileostomy and a host of other problems, has brought her husband, Ken, to the appointment—a first. They're both tall, attractive, well dressed; they seem perfectly matched.

I say to Ken, "Very glad to meet you." I'm wondering why he's here. It's a routine visit to go over Leslie's recent episode of flank pain and review her kidney stone history.

Ken shakes my hand. "Leslie always says you're great, and I thought I should say hi. We're going out to dinner afterward." He checks his watch, turns to Leslie. "Maybe you should eat some crackers? We're going to have a late supper."

"You watch out for her," I say.

Leslie rolls her eyes.

Ken says, "I do!"

"Like when?" she says.

"Like the movies, I always buy candy. And I have trail mix for plane rides. And when I make fajitas for dinner—it's low cal—I always make sure she has dessert later so she won't bottom out."

Leslie laughs. "Okay, I'll give him that. But he doesn't really consider it his job to notice when I'm low. That's up to me."

"True," he says. "I don't hover."

"I wouldn't let him anyway."

"True again." He smiles.

"It irritates me when people worry about my blood sugar or the cancer or whatever it is. I want to say, 'Back off.'"

Ken nods. "She'd already had the surgery when we met, and she always took care of her stuff on her own. The hospital's different. I go with her when she has blockages, and I went with her for the breast cancer things. But those are contained events. I think, 'Good, that's over,' and we move on."

Leslie says, "Ken's like me, he has a short attention span."

"It's not like we don't take care of each other. If she has a cold, I make her soup, and if I have one, she makes me tea. That sort of thing. But I don't think of her as sick."

Leslie, who bills herself as an impostor, has a husband who is on board with pretending. Couples sometimes collude in denying that one of them is ill, a form of shared delusion, but my sense is that the Snows aren't totally deluding themselves. They pay intermittent attention to Leslie's many troubles, but they are both more than happy to let it all go when her health doesn't demand an immediate response. Together Leslie and Ken maintain a space for normalcy. In my experience, one of the most difficult issues for families is the intrusiveness of a family member's illness—its impingement on daily life, and its interference with the growth and development of everyone in the family. By jointly believing in Leslie's quasi-fictional health, the couple make room for the ordinary pleasures (and even the ordinary pains) of living. When Leslie feels like griping, she'll complain, oh, my hip hurts, my tooth hurts, my appliance hurts. Her ileostomy appliance just goes on the list, one more mundane irritation no different from the rest.

As for her kids, they're not even sure exactly what's wrong with her. In some families, illness freezes normal development and individual growth. Young adult children, instead of launching out into the larger world of school, jobs, and relationships, can be drawn back into their family in a way that cripples them. But Leslie's children have had no problem leaving home because their mother's illness doesn't register as a roadblock. In the story Leslie has chosen to tell, her illness is the subplot, not the main narrative. It's her sense of herself as an active, autonomous agent that allows her to live "outside" of her illness and to keep her family in the realm of healthy give-and-take.[32]

Living outside of illness is not the same thing as denial; rather than say no to the facts, it adds other sources of meaning apart from the medicalized narrative of symptoms, treatments, crises, remissions. This whole book is about finding meanings—about ways to nourish identity, creativity, and hope in the face of a sickness that invites emptiness and constriction. When I'm with patients who have essentially given up, I often think of a paraphrase of something John Donne wrote: "when life shrinks to the foot of the bed."[33] To me, it's powerfully expressive of what can happen in a sickroom when pain and fear take over. The ill person closes down, isolated inside his body, and his existence grows increasingly narrow. But a relationship can open up room for meaning and allow space to think, feel, develop. It can expand life beyond the foot of the bed. The expectations people have of each other, even the friction between them, can be a source of new learning. Collisions between points of view—unavoidable when there are two people in the room—can stimulate the "growing point" I described in the previous chapter. Growing is something that two people can do together.

Some relationships are harder to put on an equal footing, and dependency is necessarily part of the picture. Can such a couple, where one is more the giver of care and the other more the taker, still sustain liveliness and meaning?

The Ungers, a ninety-year-old father and his sixty-year-old daughter, both look exhausted. Outings have become very hard for them since he's become wheelchair-dependent.

"How have your blood sugars been?" I ask. I'm wondering if he needs a little something to eat right now; he looks pale, sweaty, sleepy.

There's a silence. "Dad, did you hear what the doctor said?" Elaine bends close to her father, who sits slumped in his wheelchair.

Gerald Unger's face is almost expressionless. Among his many ailments, he has Parkinson's: the disease itself can lead to immobility, as can the medications used to treat it. What goes on inside is hard to read.

Dr. Unger says to me, "What do you know about glycine?"

He's an emeritus professor of biochemistry, long retired from teaching, but his knowledge of basic physiology and metabolism is still pretty much intact. Probably he's interested in glycine, an amino acid involved in tissue repair and blood sugar regulation, as a supplement to stave off hypoglycemia. Elaine reports that her father says "I'm dying" whenever his blood sugar plummets. He's particularly frightened when he goes to bed at night that he'll die in his sleep.

Glycine can be converted to glucose, and consequently could be useful in treating low blood sugar, but I'm not ready to recommend it. "Let me read up on glycine," I say to Dr. Unger. "For now, maybe we can tinker with your diet."

"Tinker?" Dr. Unger says. He looks disoriented.

In one of our phone conversations, Elaine told me that a previous doctor had said to her, right in front of her dad, that he was "obviously demented." Certainly he has a number of conditions that could derail him cognitively, especially given his age. Besides the Parkinson's, the hypoglycemia, and the chronic kidney disease, he's had a leg amputated because of gangrene and required cardiac catheterization to treat his atherosclerosis. His sight is failing, his hearing isn't as good as it was. It's not unlikely that his mind has slipped a notch or two. But I don't think Dr. Unger is demented. I think he has states that veer between clarity and confusion, and emotions that fluctuate according to the time of day, his dose of Parkinson's medication, his glucose level, and the daily difficulties of just trying to live.

I look at Dr. Unger's blank face; I know better than to assume his mind is empty. I tell him that at bedtime he should drink a "slurry"—a concoction of water and cornstarch that the body metabolizes slowly over time. "It will see you through the night."

Elaine reaches over to her father and squeezes his arm. "You can have it with your coconut cream pie." She turns to me. "It's his favorite. He has it almost every night before he goes to bed."

I smile at Dr. Unger. "Sounds delicious."

Dr. Unger shrugs. His face is still masklike, but I see, or imagine, a gleam in his eyes.

The Ungers represent another kind of couple that come to my office: an elderly patient with an adult child. More often than not, the child is a daughter. There are, of course, exceptions. One son I know routinely accompanies his elderly mother to all her many doctor appointments, keeps track of all her labs, and emails her physicians with updates on her condition. But caregiving in families still tends to fall to women—the classical "nurturers"—rather than men. Elaine and her father are unusually attuned. She knows what he wants even when he's having trouble with words, and she is patient with the storms of irrationality that sometimes overtake him. In a sense, she's motherly toward him.

Such a role reversal is common with adult children and their aging parents. Children become maternal, or paternal, toward the parents who raised them. How this intergenerational dependence works out is a complex business, influenced by individual temperament and history. When things haven't gone so well in the past, adult children may refuse responsibility for parents they feel were indifferent to them, and aging parents may refuse the grudging care of disgruntled offspring. But even if family ties are strong, it may not be easy. One elderly woman I know confided to me that she worries all the time about how her illness is affecting her daughter. "She has no life," the woman told me. "I hate it that I'm doing this to her." But the daughter told me, "This is the most meaningful thing I could ever do. I think our culture is too hard on families. It's as though the only way to make it in America is to be totally separate and independent. What's wrong with loving and caring for each other? What's wrong with being close?"

Close relationships often contain the seeds of regression and dependency. Are those things "wrong"? In the case of the very old, it seems just to make room for the expression of ultimate needs. We begin life dependent on those who love us, and there is symmetry, even a kind of beauty, when life ends that way. This isn't to say that relationships between the old and their grownup children are always of the Hallmark variety. Feelings run high even in the best of families: sometimes caregivers feel strangled by too many demands, and elderly parents feel demeaned or guilty. Those who don't turn to family can also have a rough time. Aging parents who sidestep their children and seek care in nursing homes have to find connections that in some sense substitute for their personal relationships, and that's often a thorny task. But connections are vital, maybe especially so as life wanes and expectations fade. Without other people, life ends before it ends.

Helen Rosen, eighty-seven, suffering from spinal stenosis and chronic kidney disease, is sitting hunched over in her wheelchair, her bright blond hair pouffed in a do. She's come from the nursing home with Velma, her aide, who hovers close by.

Helen is explaining how you get good care in a nursing home. This is a tricky business, as I've learned from others who are in assisted living. Some of the older patients I see are prickly with their aides, and vice versa. These patients never wanted to move to a home, and they detest the impersonal care they receive; meanwhile, the aides seem annoyed with the slowness and incapacity (and sometimes the ill temper) of the people in their charge.

Helen says, "The people who don't get on don't know how to do it."

"How do you do it?"

"First off," she says, touching Velma's arm, "I hired Velma. My daughter tried to get me someone, but that one was always saying, what can I get for you, what should I do next. But I didn't want a maid. Velma is a friend."

Velma smiles.

"She comes three times a week, and we go out together. She always fig-ures out the best way to do things. She can see the forest for the trees. Also, we're very polite together. I say, 'Can I get you a glass of water?' and she says, 'Yes, thank you.' I think manners are very important between people."

Velma, meanwhile, is still smiling. "She's forgetting how much she gives me," she says. "I'm blessed to know someone like her."

"Oh, phoo," Helen says, but Velma nods: yes, it's true.

"What about the other staff?" I ask.

Helen steeples her fingers. "Well, I consider their point of view. I never ask for help unless it's strictly necessary, and I think they appreciate that. I don't know why other people can't be more patient—I can't stand the ones who complain all the time. Of course, to be fair, I wanted to go into the home, and a lot of people didn't. And my daughters visit me, which is helpful."

"And when you're in pain?"

"I just wait. Someone will come eventually."

Helen understands that the connection between caregiver and ill person isn't strictly business, founded on money and defined by hours of work. It's a relationship, and an intimate one. At the nursing home, she has drawn on her innate politeness and her awareness of other people to forge solid connections with caregivers. But it's still Velma, a personal friend, who matters most. Velma helps her with her body, maneuvering the walker and the wheelchair, doing the driving, taking her mind off her pain. But there's also give-and-take: Helen treats Velma to lunch, Velma brings Helen fresh flowers, and when they go on errands, it's an adventure. Helen says her sense of humor disappeared after the death of her husband, but

Velma has brought it back. Velma, who never did a puzzle in her life before, says Helen has turned her into a crossword addict.

The relationship is a growing point. The two of them expect things of each other, and, in rising to meet each other's vision, they change. Sometimes when people are sick, others are afraid to ask things of them, tiptoeing carefully in deference to the ill one's greater needs. But this apparent delicacy is really only a form of retreat. When the sick person is invited to take over all the space, he loses the opportunity to bump into a different point of view and another set of needs and expectations. And it's only by sharing, ex-pecting—even, at times, struggling—that two people can help each other grow and develop.

"Can I ask you a question?" Leonard asks for the fourth time. His office visits are always like this, with a refrain of questions running through. He has schizophrenia, and there's a certain off-kilter quality to the conversa-tion: his questions are often tangential to the issue at hand. He's close to forty, and after years of antipsychotic medication, he has serious diabetes and renal shutdown. But he doesn't want to know about any of that. He wants to know if his urine is "wrong," if he can drink soda, if I plan on taking any blood.

This last point is, as it were, a sticking point. He's refused dialysis be-cause of all the needles, and now he's asking if the transplant he's waiting for will require any blood draws.

George, his aide, raises his eyebrows at me. George knows everything about Leonard's way of doing things—what you can say to him, what you'd better skip. Logic is not Leonard's strong suit, so reminding him that he has blood draws all the time to check his lipid profile and to make sure he hasn't developed agranulocytosis on clozapine, his antipsychotic medication, will get me nowhere.

I say, "Can I ask you a question?"

Leonard laughs. He has an excellent sense of humor. "Sure."

"Can I schedule the blood work so you can get your new kidney?"

Who knows why this works? But Leonard says, "Sure."

With Leonard, I don't go into long-winded explanations of things; I take him as he is. When he refused dialysis, I didn't hammer home that he would die without it—a logic that he didn't care to, or couldn't, follow. Instead I arranged to have a transplant specialist talk to him. And when he came back to see me with "Can I ask you a question?" I let him ask away until it was my turn to ask him a question. In the end, he agreed to the transplant and asked if I'd visit him during his hospital stay. It was somewhat unusual for me to make that kind of visit, because I'm not the transplant physician, but of course I went. He greeted me with, "Can I ask you a question?" and we both laughed.

George deserves a lot of the credit for Leonard's good outcome. For people with chronic mental illness, the caregiver has immense importance. A caregiver—family member, aide, life coach, roommate—who is strongly present and involved helps steady the course of a person who suffers from disruptions in consciousness, attention, and mood. Such a companion can be like an "extra mind," lending context and continuity to someone who is often at sea. In the course of appointments, Leonard would often check George's face for reassurance; George, at the same time, would be subtly helping the conversation along. When Leonard asked if he could delay the transplant until after his birthday, George signaled "yes," and I quickly agreed. Privately, George told me to indicate the date of the transplant only a short time before the operation, to spare Leonard intolerable anxiety. He glued things together for Leonard and smoothed the way for me.

In a way, George and Leonard represent an extreme case, not unlike the Ungers, in that Leonard's difficulties required George to take on the greater responsibility. He was more the giver, Leonard more the taker. The two illustrate what can happen when people lean on people: Leonard could go forward and do something unimaginable, because George was there to help him imagine it. George and Leonard shouldered the burden of Leonard's difficult life between them.

What makes someone shoulder another's burden? To take another extreme case, what would make someone want to donate an organ to another person?

Daniel and Ginny are sitting across from me, holding hands. This couple is in it together, as I've come to know from our monthly meetings over two years.

I clear my throat, and I can tell Ginny knows even before I speak. "It's time," I say.

Daniel looks blank. He's not on top of it like Ginny, even though he's just been telling me how much worse it's been lately. They've been living in the North End after a move from their hometown in New Hampshire (Ginny calls it "a third world country" when it comes to medicine), and she and Daniel have been walking to his appointments, a long trek across downtown Boston to the Brigham. That walk, very important to Daniel— a sign that "I can still do it"—has become harder and harder. Another thing that's kept him in the game is lunch with Ginny at North End restaurants—wonderful Italian food—every day at two o'clock; but that, too, is getting harder to do. (Ginny says, "And I've gained twenty pounds. But it's worth it.") Lately Daniel has been dragging himself up the stairs to the apartment at six-thirty or seven in the evening, and going straight to bed. The trips back to New Hampshire once a week, to keep an eye on the adult hockey league he runs, have become impossible, even though it's Ginny who drives. And he's getting very forgetful, from "Where did I put the keys?" to his brother's telephone number.

"It's time," I say again.

"Time for what?" Daniel asks.

"Dialysis or transplant." I leave out the third thing, but I can see Ginny register what I've omitted: or death.

The Adelsons have a strong marriage that represents the best kind of optimism and resilience. Their relationship illustrates how much the presence of another can help a person find meaning beyond, even within, illness. But as we'll see, their story is ultimately about two couples; not just husband and wife but also recipient and donor. Because Daniel received his transplant from an unrelated donor, his experience illuminates another kind of bond, forged between two people of their own free will, without the facilitating element of family obligation.

The story begins with Daniel going for a routine vasectomy, where the doctor discovered a blood pressure so high that he wouldn't let Daniel leave the hospital without a kidney consult and an immediate ultrasound. Daniel got the phone call that night: he had polycystic kidney disease, the same genetic disease that Tom Mahon, the amateur genealogist, had. Daniel says "shock" doesn't begin to describe how he felt. His mother, Leah, who'd had PKD for decades and had been on dialysis for years, had told him that it affected only the women in a family. (His grandmother and aunt also had PKD, so on the face of it, gender seemed to be the decisive factor.) Now Daniel was in despair: having watched his mother struggle with her illness since he was a teenager, he felt his future disappearing. He was convinced that he'd never be able to live on dialysis. He was an active guy, an athlete. Life on a machine was not for him.

Ginny's reaction was fury about the secrets and lies in her husband's family. She'd asked Leah, before the wedding, if there was any chance Daniel would get the disease, and Leah had told her the same thing she'd told Daniel: only women. When Ginny confronted her with Daniel's diagnosis, Leah said, "Well, that's what I always thought. You should have looked into it more." Leah's longtime dialysis doctor regretted that he hadn't insisted everyone in the family get tested long ago. Meanwhile, Ginny had their daughters, then ages two and four, evaluated right away: both turned out to have PKD. This "crashed down" on Daniel, as Ginny puts it; he had carried the bad gene to his daughters. Ginny, too, was devastated for a long period. Over time, though, Ginny made peace with the facts and even forgave her mother-in-law. With some self-reflection (and a little help from a marriage counselor), she came to understand denial not as a lie but an attempt to fend off painful realities.

Fortunately, Daniel was asymptomatic for a long time after the diagnosis. A New Hampshire nephrologist tracked his creatinine and prescribed antihypertensives. When I talk to Daniel about his illness, he always says the same thing: "I could take anything, but I was worried about what it was doing to my wife and daughters." Through a period of ten years or more, as his kidney function slowly declined, his chief concern was to hide his symptoms from his family. He wouldn't talk about his increasing fatigue and weakness, and just kept working at the rink: up at five in the morning, going in on weekends and holidays, and even continuing to play hockey himself. He tried to show up for all the girls' school events and stay involved with his family, regardless of what else was going on.

It was when Daniel's creatinine began to rise above 2—a sure sign that his kidneys were failing to excrete waste products in the urine—that he came to see me, moving from New Hampshire to the North End to be closer to the Brigham. Only then did Daniel let go of his self-sufficiency ("the guy thing," Ginny calls it) and allow himself to lean more on Ginny. For the next two years, I helped Daniel stave off the end of renal function; meanwhile, injections of erythropoietin, which helped generate red blood cells in his own circulation, improved his sense of well-being, at least temporarily.

When the couple began actively to search for an organ donor, sending out feelers in every direction, Ginny says the outpouring of generosity was amazing: the phone rang off the wall. In the close-knit community of the New Hampshire hockey league, thirty people signed up to be tested. Most were over the age of forty, which meant, Daniel says, that something or other was wrong with them, because everyone begins to have health issues by then. A typical example was his oldest brother: the only sibling to have escaped the genetic curse of PKD, he was ruled out because of kidney stones. Others were ineligible because, even if their blood type was compatible, there was a tissue or immunologic mismatch.

The story to this point charts a familiar journey: the shock of diagnosis, the search for a cause (devolving, at times, into blame), the struggle to live "outside" the illness, the mutual protectiveness of family members. Daniel had arrived at a narrative crux, the dialysis-or-else moment, when things took a surprising turn. A friend in the hockey league, Hank Reston, took Daniel out to lunch; he'd noticed that Daniel had stopped showing up at the rink, and asked why. Daniel explained that he had end-stage renal disease, and Hank promptly said, "I'll give you a kidney." Hank is chief financial officer of a major food franchise, famous in his part of the world and liked by everyone; coming from a large Catholic family (ten siblings), he joked, "I have my donors all lined up in case I get into any trouble." Miraculously, Hank was a perfect match, and the transplant went forward. They still joke about it. Daniel will say, "Your kidney was pretty good—now can I have your liver?" Hank, when they're out on the ice together, will yell at Daniel, "Stay away from me! I only have one kidney!"

Daniel is, in fact, still on the ice, and with the blessing of his transplant doctor, who gave him the following advice: (1) avoid large risks (specifically, don't play with people you don't know), (2) live your life, (3) protect yourself. A friend of Daniel's in the pro shop built him special protective gear for his new kidney, which Daniel describes as a "little lump" that you can see under the skin of his abdomen. (Transplants go in the front instead of the back, where the kidney would normally be found.) The protection consists of a goalie's shoulder pad sewn into a girdle that protects his lower torso: he could get hit with a slap shot and be fine.

The transplant was a complete success. Daniel's doctor has told him that, looking at his lab values, no one would ever know he didn't have his own kidneys. The immunosuppressive medication hasn't been a problem, and Daniel feels great. "It really is the gift of life," he says. "I've had to struggle a little, because I'm not one to ask or take anything from anyone. And how do you repay a person for something like that?" I asked what he thought had motivated Hank, and he said Hank always quotes Saint Augustine: "Since you cannot do good to all, you are to pay special attention to those who, by accidents of time, or place, or circumstance, are brought into closer connection with you."

The sense of connection between the two men has continued for the last several years, with an annual picnic on Memorial Day, close to the anniversary of the transplant, to celebrate the event. Daniel says that at a recent picnic, he gave Hank a framed picture of the two of them with the caption "To my brother, who gave me life." He says it's been hard for him because what Hank did is so enormous, a debt you can't erase; he broke down in tears when he handed Hank the photograph. But Hank says he's the one who's grateful. It made his life meaningful to give life to someone else.

Daniel's story underscores that both the giver and the taker gain; that their roles are, in a sense, reversible. He who gives, gets; he who gets, gives. All the pairs I've described here—the married ones but also the other couples—have expanded their lives by sharing the burden of illness. An ill person needs a partner not only to provide care or help but to open up a space of possibility; a space for sharing, enrichment, growth. The back-and-forth of a close relationship staves off the loneliness of living inside a body that doesn't work right; offers solace for the pain of bad luck and hard times; and, even when illness threatens to narrow the prospect of the future, nourishes playfulness, liveliness, and hope. But such a relationship doesn't only benefit the one who's sick. Both partners are transformed. Both partners, coming up against each other, waking up to each other's point of view, grow together toward the future.

⌒

It's after dinner, before dessert, and my wife is doing that thing I hate, her thumb pushing the imaginary plunger on an insulin syringe. I flick her an "okay" and grope under the tablecloth for my pump, then surreptitiously punch in a few units and stick it back in my pants pocket. "There," I say with my eyes, "satisfied?"

She nods primly: thank you very much.

It's so irritating. Why doesn't she just leave it to me?

But I know the answer to that: without her little thumb thing, I would undoubtedly have let it go until I got home, and then my glucose would have been superhigh. And I would have been hot and bothered, the way I get when my sugar is over the top, and we might have had words. She's saving the day, for me and for her.

And I remember, too, that she's there when the opposite is occurring, when my glucose is plunging and the world is going dim. I don't have to tell her, she's just on it, slipping me Life Savers as the lights go down in the theater or handing me a Coke from her backpack when we're traipsing in the woods. She knows from looking at me, my skin flushed or pale, my hand fluttering to the back of my head, a tone in my voice or something in my gait—all kinds of things. The way we play these moments out has become a private theme, a way of being in it together; as I'm in it with her too, I hope, when she needs help.

I think back to my very first appointment with the diabetologist, decades ago, when I asked if my wife could give me insulin injections. He told me, "You have to do this alone." Yes, but as it's turned out, not completely alone. I've had good company.

Conclusion: Bluefish

Rick, my neighbor, is outside cleaning up his yard. We've had a tough winter in Boston, one big snowstorm after another, and limbs and branches litter the lawn. The flowerbeds are matted with dry leaves, but I see that his crocuses, pale purple and yellow, are already poking up.

I comment on the early flowers.

"The flowers are Nan's department. I'm just the hired hand," he says.

"How are you feeling these days?" I ask.

"The colostomy's been great! I was having blockages, so everything would back up and then all of a sudden let loose. It was wearing me out. I have a lot more energy now. Nan says I'm like a new person."

"What made you decide to go ahead with it?" I wonder what I would do if it were me.

"It's no picnic—the appliance is tricky, and, unfortunately, the colostomy nurses were all women. You'd think I'd enjoy that, but not under the circumstances. There I am with my pants off, up to my elbows in shit, and

they're pointing like airline stewardesses showing how the seat belt works. 'This flap goes here.'"

We laugh.

"Mainly I figured it out myself. Really, I should write a how-to manual. But I'll say this, it's a lot better than what I was having before. Talk about a mess." Rick shrugs, smiles. "I figure I can tell it like it is with you. You're a doctor."

I do feel privileged to know a lot of truths that are kept hidden from others. I remember my dad, when I said I wanted to be a doctor, telling me that it was a big job. Patients would tell me their deepest secrets. I would see them naked in body and soul.

I tell Rick that I'm glad he's better.

"Much better. I was up in New Hampshire a month ago, and I skied a black diamond trail."

"Black diamond?"

"They're the steepest runs, really challenging. I haven't been able to take one of the hard trails for years now. You know, Nan says I'm a new person, but what I feel is, I'm back to myself. I'm the same person I was. A slightly older version, but still me."

I've come back to Rick, whom you met in the introduction, to look deeper into his story—a success story that involves more than the fact that he's alive and doing better. In the course of a number of run-ins with illness, he's dug down inside for reserves of strength and habits of mind that have helped him bounce back over and over again. As he says, "It's never going away—I'll always be 'sick.'" He's referring not only to the type 2 diabetes that emerged when he was about fifty but to the cancers he's had. They haven't killed him, but they've carved up his body, sapped his energy, and forced him to face the specter of death.

Even though treatments have gotten better, you can't hear the word *cancer* without thinking "death." Rick says that, by comparison, diabetes hardly registered on his radar. He takes his oral medication and tests his sugars twice a day; but apart from a little fatigue and some attention to diet (handled mostly by Nan, his wife and manager-in-chief), his late-onset diabetes hasn't made a huge difference in his life. But cancer, Rick says, was a "holy shit" moment. He thought, "No way, they've got the wrong guy." Even so, when he was diagnosed six years ago, he didn't think all that much about dying. He was too preoccupied with the practicalities of having a tumor in his colon. He'd never had an operation in his life, and he had to gear up for major surgery involving the removal of part of his colon and most of his rectum. He had to deal with the postsurgical pain. He had to deal with unpleasant physical consequences. (Things like occasional incontinence are not, he says, "a total pleasure.")

Generally speaking, Rick was busy coping with the thing immediately in front of him and forgetting the thing just past. "I live in squares of time," he says. "My mind's like that." For one thing, he's a computer programmer and systems analyst, good at calculating probabilities and determining what he can, and can't, solve. The things he can't fix, he puts aside. Also, he had what he calls a "screwed up" childhood, with an abusive alcoholic father. Although he blames his younger brother's emotional troubles and early death on the trauma of their rearing, for Rick the bad childhood had a different effect: it conditioned him to block out the bad stuff and focus on the art of the possible. You could say that he has a gift for forgetting, which, you'll remember, is one of the coping strategies outlined in this book.

A tour of Rick's medical history illustrates the other seven strategies too. For example, be yourself. Rick says he learned from the bad childhood to never let anyone else, or anything else, define him. "Illness isn't who I am. It's why I can mention the cancer and the colostomy to people without feeling bad about it. Nan always says, 'Don't tell them,' but I think, 'Why not?' I certainly don't think of myself as my colostomy. Why should they? Of course, they do, sometimes. People hear 'cancer,' and they think, 'It could happen to me.' But that's more their problem than mine."

He's also been able to handle treatment with a fairly good grace, and to accept limitations when necessary. He hasn't fallen into the trap of being "too sick" or "not sick." In the language I've been using, he knows himself, which allows him to be "just sick enough." Rick says, "People can overfocus and 'create' the disease. But Nan wasn't going to let me carry on and whine and collapse. She was always saying, 'Get your ass out of bed.' She also made sure I went in for checkups and that I didn't run away from things. And I was lucky in my doctor. Nan worked for Dr. Feldman back when she was in high school and college, and he's like a family friend. He doesn't take any guff from me—he doesn't overdo the 'You're okay,' but he also says, 'Get going.' He calls up to ask how I am and keeps tabs on me. So I walk the line pretty well."

About a year after his colon surgery, Rick lost his job at the computer firm he'd helped found. It had been sold to a larger conglomerate, and the powers-that-be decided he'd lost some of his edge since his illness. Getting fired was a blow to his ego, but over time he came to terms with it. Rick found out he liked not working. He kept busy with household projects and got more involved in helping kids. Years ago he'd volunteered at a Boys and Girls Club north of Boston, but now there were his own children: two from his first marriage and one with Nan. The older two were launching careers and getting married, while his youngest son was still in high school.

When Eric finally left for college, Nan's fifteen-year-old learning-disabled niece came to live with them. Now Rick was busy all over again with school conferences and chauffeuring. This latest phase of parenting was, to use the language of the book, an opportunity to transform and grow. And a late-arriving gift, a new grandchild born to his daughter last winter, has given him a literal "growing point." Rick says Deirdre Rose is his reward for persevering.

Rick was beginning to feel he had his life back. Even though he knew he'd never be "normal," he felt confident he wasn't going to die, and his days had a rhythm that made sense. But then, three or four years after the colon cancer, Rick got his next diagnosis: prostate cancer. This turned out to be a very big deal. The radiation treatments of years before had turned his insides to "mush." (Rick wryly notes this was the "technical" term that the doctors used.) As Rick understands it, his urethra was fused to his prostate, so any attempt to operate would destroy the urethra, which, the doctors told him, would be "a very bad outcome." Rick took that as code for "you're cooked": if there were no way for his body to excrete urine, he'd die. Two different surgeons, both experts in prostate cancer, refused to operate on him except as a "last resort."

It was around then that Rick began having middle-of-the-night thoughts. He'd look up at the ceiling and think about headstones and what it would be like to meet his Maker. He says he was raised Catholic, but he's casual about it; he and Nan go to the church that's around the corner mainly "because it's there." But he believes in God; not the details of any one religion, necessarily, but a principle or force that underlies the mysteries of an infinite universe. ("You could say I believe in *dis*organized religion.") Sometimes, as a residue of his upbringing, Rick gets nervous about heaven and "the other place," but mainly he's made his peace with uncertainty. He says we can't know what happens after we die: one place, the other place, or maybe just nothing. We have to accept our unknowingness.

During those sleepless nights, he came a long way to accepting his mortality. "Everybody dies some time." He didn't feel the need to run into the church; he wasn't the best Catholic in the history of the world. But at fifty-nine, he could say he'd done some good in his life, particularly his work with young people. He could say he'd had wonderful experiences, wonderful relationships, and he'd accomplished some things. It wasn't as though he were thirty and just starting out. He could say he'd lived.

In the terms I've been using, Rick was able to transcend his physical hardships and find solace and acceptance through his personal brand of faith. He could also forgive himself. He had some bad moments—"What did I do to deserve this? Why am I being punished?"—but, in the end, he concluded his prostate disease was just bad luck.

But then the world offered him a surprise. He got a referral to a cryosurgeon, a man specializing in a technique for freezing necrotic tissues and tumor cells. Dr. Bradshaw was a jokester who reminded Rick of Nan's cousin Peter: LOL funny, but also totally nuts. Could he be for real? Dr. Bradshaw spent the first twenty minutes telling jokes, his hands flying all over, and then as an aside mentioned that Rick would be in and out of the hospital in twenty-four hours, which turned out to be accurate. The tumor got zapped, the urethra was intact. Rick felt like he'd dodged death.

Rick feels lucky, "given the alternative," but life still hasn't been easy. An accomplished skier, he got back on his skis not long after the cryosurgery and, five hundred yards down an easy slope, slipped at three miles an hour on a patch of ice and broke his hip—which meant four months on crutches and in a wheelchair to avoid putting weight on the fractured bone. This was a setback not only to his body but his pride. And he wasn't finished with set-backs: his malabsorption problems and intestinal blockages, persisting after his colon surgery of years ago, finally pushed him to have the colostomy. And he still wears "man diapers" to deal with urinary incontinence left over from the prostate cancer.

The hip, the colostomy, the diapers—none of these things, Rick claims, is much of a problem. But it's clear, despite the bravado, that these things occasionally *are* a problem. He's half-irritated, half-offended, that people back off when he's too frank about the details of his physical condition. The stoma, the surgically created opening where the bowel has been redirected, is above his belt line, and he worries about clothing. Sometimes he's anxious about spills and smells emanating from the bag. But he tries to get past his bad moments and usually arrives at a better state. The way he puts it: "I tend to round off the negatives." He's happy to have his energy back. He forgets. He moves on. He is who he is, no apologies.

This past winter, his friend Steven called him up and said, "You're doing this"—going back to the mountain where he fell. Steve made all the arrangements, and there Rick was, looking down the slope from the top of the trail; not just any trail but a black dia-mond one, steep, with sharp twists and turns. This was the test of being better. He felt nervous but not as afraid as he thought he'd be. Then he shoved off, and it was like always: like flying. He thought he'd do it just once, to prove he could, but he immediately wanted to do it again. "It was a rush. It gave me back my body."

Most of all, Rick has Nan. She's his cheerleader and coach, his efficiency expert and fan club, and a devout believer in "you can do it." Rick admits he has his moments of depression and self-pity, but one reason the bad moments don't last long is Nan, with her no-nonsense encouragement. "She's my true primary caregiver." He thinks of her as his better half, but they're also a good team. He ignores, she pays attention. He's a fatalist, she's an activist. He feels bad, she says, "That's enough." He lets himself depend on her care, and she thrives on giving.

At least that's how Rick tells it. But he says I should really talk to Nan, who might have a different view. I already know Nan a little from over-the-fence conversations, and her briskness and clarity are refreshing. I imagine (and, indeed, Rick has told me) that her acerbic take on things effectively curtails his periodic lapses into self-indulgence. It's not all sugar candy next door; there's some salt and vinegar in the mix. At least from over the fence, their marriage looks like one of those good partnerships I talked about in the previous chapter, where the collisions are fruitful and one person's expectations help the other one grow.

This may all seem like paint by numbers, Rick's life as a checklist of coping mechanisms. The point is, with chronic illness, you need everything you've got. The maxims I've listed point to the paradox at the heart of the stories in this book. Illness represents a hard limit—an unyielding reality that closes off possibility, compromises freedom, undermines desire and hope. At the same time, being sick opens up unexpected opportunities for creativity and growth. By taking away the "taken-for-granted," illness invites, even forces, new awareness and new learning. By exploring parts of the self that were once hidden by everyday routine, a sick person can find his way to creative expression, personal transformation, emotional enrichment. And though being sick is hard, very hard (ask Rick; ask anyone), it's not the end of playfulness and joy. In the spirit of the ancients, we can play seriously, *serio ludere,* as we do battle with our illnesses.

In Rick's case, though his traumatic childhood undoubtedly haunts him, it also gave him the capacity to set things aside, keep going, adapt. All of us who suddenly have to face an illness can discover within ourselves capacities like these. Facing up to adversity is less a matter of deciding to be strong than of letting go and seeing what comes next. What is most required in order to thrive "after the diagnosis" is the capacity to stay open to experience. By letting life happen and time go forward, we can hold on to future hopes and present meanings. We can find our way to "next." We can find our way to "now."

It's August in East Hampton, one of those end-of-summer days, and we're heading out into Three Mile Harbor in the skiff. Sometimes I fish alone, and my wife packs me sandwiches and Coke in case my blood sugar gets low when I'm out in the middle of nowhere. Today we're together, which means I don't have to think about it. She's my infrastructure; not always a good thing, for her or for me, but today I'm just happy that I can concentrate on fishing.

We dump the life jackets, the food, the bait, and the rods into the boat. I check the gas and oil, rev the engine. My wife casts off.

We discuss whether we should go down the harbor to the Sound. Going the length of it takes a while, because you have to go slow, "No Wake," as the sign says, and there might be whitecaps on the Sound. The skiff isn't built for big seas.

While we talk it over, I've got a rod trailing in the water. My wife starts looking up. "Hey," she says.

"What?"

"Look."

She points skyward. I can't see much, just some moving flecks of black and white, but I can hear them: terns. Their ragged cries come and go.

She describes what she's seeing: the terns are beginning to cluster in one spot near the deep-water channel at the center of the harbor. The wind picks up, the noise picks up. I maneuver the skiff into the channel, and now the birds are close enough for me to make out. They're swirling, screaming, plunging. The water foams. Bursts of spray shoot up. Bluefish are breaking the surface, chasing glass minnows that flash silver in the water. There's a tug on my rod, and I pull in a nice one, unhook it, throw the line back in, and immediately catch another. The fish flop in the bottom of the boat, spitting bait.

My wife tucks her feet under her, away from the teeth. Blues can bite.

I hand her the rod, and as she's protesting that she doesn't know how to fish, I watch her feel the tug and pull one in.

We stop when the baitfish begin to move farther down the harbor. The whole show—flashing minnows, splashing blues, screaming terns—continues farther off. I lose sight of them quickly. "They're over there," my wife says, gesturing, but it's just a smudge to me.

We sit quietly, shoulder to shoulder, listening to the water lap against the boat.

After a while, we motor toward the marina at the head of the harbor. I drop anchor in an inlet away from the main channel, pull out my fillet knife, and begin to gut and scale the carcasses. We've caught fifteen, enough to feed the crowd back at the house.

The light glances off the water, the colors glow. It's perfect.

My wife always thinks I'm too optimistic about fishing. She'll say, "What makes you think they're lining up under there? What are the odds?" She's more of a pessimist, or maybe a realist.

But she's smiling now. I smile back. I feel happy, fish piled up at my feet, the two of us in the same boat.

Acknowledgments

I want to express my deep gratitude to the following people—
"without whom, nothing":

My patients, who shared with me the meanings they found in illness and motivated the writing of this book.

My teachers, especially Milford Fulop, who shaped my understanding of disease, diagnosis, and treatment.

My colleague Dr. Susan Carlson at Mt. Edgecumbe Hospital, who
hosted the field trip to Sitka, Alaska.

Two Harvard PhD students who contributed case materials: Valerie LeBleu, for the polycystic kidney disease story (Tom Mahon)
described in chapter 2; and Cherie Lynn Ramirez, for the osteomalacia story (Juan Golardo) described in chapter 4.

Two readers, Mark O'Connell and Laurie Raymond, whose sensi-
tive insights deepened my thinking.

My literary "attendings":

Paul Bresnick, my agent, wise in a domain I knew nothing about,
whose energy and enthusiasm made this book a reality.

Sydny Miner, my first editor, whose excellent judgment and crisp editing benefited the manuscript enormously.

Michelle Rorke, who took over the reins after Sydny, and whose dedication and hard work carried the project over the finish line.

My wife and collaborator, Betsy, who has been by my side year after year, through calm waters and rough seas, in the same boat.

Bibliography

Fadiman, Anne. *The Spirit Catches You and You Fall Down: A Hmong Child, Her American Doctors, and the Collision of Two Cultures* (New York: Farrar, Straus & Giroux, 1997).

Groopman, Jerome. *How Doctors Think* (Boston: Houghton Mifflin, 2007).

LeDoux, Joseph. *The Emotional Brain: The Mysterious Underpinnings of Emotional Life* (New York: Simon & Schuster, 1998).

Metcalfe, Peter. *Gumboot Determination: The Story of the SouthEast Alaska Regional Health Consortium* (SEARHC, 2005).

Pories, Susan, MD, Sachin Jain, and Gordon Harper, MD, eds. *The Soul of a Doctor: Harvard Medical Students Face Life and Death* (Chapel Hill, NC: Algonquin Books, 2006).

Sapolsky, Robert. *Why Zebras Don't Get Ulcers: The Acclaimed Guide to Stress, Stress-Related Diseases, and Coping* (New York: Henry Holt, 1998).

Schachter, Daniel L., *The Seven Sins of Memory: How the Mind Forgets and Remembers* (Boston and New York: Houghton Mifflin, 2001).

Notes

Chapter 1: Doctor-Patient 101

1. The divide between doctors and patients is a recurrent theme in *The Soul of a Doctor: Harvard Medical Students Face Life and Death,* a collection of essays written by Harvard Medical students about their indoctrination into the profession. Many students describe their struggle to sustain a feeling of connection with the person in the bed when their job almost demands some distance.

2. Dr. Katharine Treadway, an associate professor of medicine at Harvard Medical School, tries to inculcate empathy in Patient-Doctor 2, the second-year course that teaches history taking and physical examination by telling stories about real patients. "I think of these stories as tiny vaccines against the loss of compassion that comes from the overwhelming tasks of clinical clerkships, from long hours fraught with anxiety about performing well, about getting the right diagnosis, the right treatment plans, about mastering an enormous amount of knowledge . . . I hope these vaccinations will remind them during the long nights ahead that there is always a person attached to the disease and that giving comfort is one of their fundamental tasks." *New England Journal of Medicine,* vol. 352, no. 19 (May 12, 2005), p. 1943.

Chapter 2: My Name Is Lucy Rooney

3. Rachel Sobel, in her essay "MSL—Medicine as a Second Language," writes, "In one respect, the classroom years were a massive vocabulary lesson in 'medicalese.' . . . Legend has it that after medical school, a newly minted doctor has some 55,000 new words in the memory bank." She notes that as a medical student on the wards, she is "charged with the task of translation. Indeed, I must constantly navigate two worlds, patient-speak and doctor-speak, and hardly do the two meet." *New England Journal of Medicine*, vol. 352, no. 19 (May 12, 2005), pp. 1945–46.

4. Dana Jennings, in a December 16, 2008, *New York Times* article entitled "Person, Patient, Statistic," writes about his fellow patients, men with prostate cancer, who sit stunned and silent in waiting rooms: "They don't understand that to keep from being a cipher, a mere 'case,' you need to be conscious and verbal. As a patient, when you don't speak . . . all you become is 'meat,' quiet meat."

5. I've noticed that when a person is diagnosed can influence his basic attitudes and adjustments; he can be stuck in the moment when he first became ill, and slow to catch up with technological advances. For diabetics, two improvements have vastly influenced self-care. Glucometers have become streamlined and finger sticks nearly painless, so that testing blood sugars is far friendlier than when I started out. And the insulin pump allows better delivery of insulin; you can infuse a slow drip over the course of the day to meet minimal metabolic requirements, and deliver larger quantities discreetly, as needed, by dialing in units on the pump, rather than clumsily filling a syringe and injecting in plain sight of everybody else. Another change in diabetes care is the newer emphasis on keeping blood sugar low. Hyperglycemia wasn't even understood to be a risk factor for complications at the time I was diagnosed, and the practice back then was to err on the side of high glucose rather than try for tight control.

6. I am indebted to Valerie LeBleu for the discussion of Tom's case as described in her unpublished report, "Tom's Polycystic Kidneys: A Mentored Clinical Case Book," Harvard Medical School, 2006–07.

7. Michener's essay, "The Dialysis Calendar, April 24, 1997," can be found online at http://nephron.com/nephsites/nic/michener.html.

Chapter 3: Too Sick. Not Sick. Just Sick Enough.

8. The number of visits to alternative medicine practitioners is cited by Theresa Schraeder in a review of Roberta Bivins's *Alternative Medicine? A History,* in the *New England Journal of Medicine,* vol. 359, no. 5 (July 31, 2008), pp. 543–44.

9. Validation sometimes depends on the country you live in. A young woman came to see me with blood in her urine and pain low in her abdomen. I told her that in England she'd be diagnosed with "loin pain hematuria," but in the United States there was no such diagnosis. (Which doesn't mean there is no such thing. I've seen several young women with this same cluster of symptoms.)

Chapter 4: More Things in Heaven and Earth

10. This chapter is about the spiritual dimension that is so often absent from discussions of patient care. "More things in heaven and earth" is a line from *Hamlet,* act 1, scene 5: Hamlet, having just seen his father's ghost, passionately tells Horatio, his classmate from Wittenberg and a confirmed skeptic, "There are more things in heaven and earth than are dreamt of in your philosophy."

11. The positive effect of belief on physical well-being has become a standard trope in our culture. From professional publications like the *Journal of Aging and Health* (source of the study on religious services) to popular magazines such as *Newsweek* (source of the study on cardiovascular risk and Seligman's views on optimism), the message is consistent: belief and optimism can promote health. I agree that they can, even if the mechanism is not entirely understood, but the inverse—that continued illness represents a failure of belief—is clearly not true. Diseases are complicated, causes uncertain, treatments unpredictable. You can applaud (and cultivate) positive thinking without blaming people for being ill.

12. The study about breast cancer (D. E. Stewart, A. M. Cheung, S. Duff, F. Wong, M. McQuestion, T. Cheng, et al., "Attributions of Cause and Recurrence in Long-Term Breast Cancer Survivors," 2001) is cited not only in a scientific review article but in a Sunday *New York Times Magazine* article—another instance of how deeply the notion of positive thinking is embedded in the popular consciousness.

13. I am indebted to Harvard PhD candidate Cherie Lynn Ramirez for her write-up of this case of osteomalacia (2008), which helped me recall the chronology of events.

Chapter 5: Who Will I Be Today?

14. The transformations achieved by Cassandra, Leslie, and other patients of mine owe something to the mind's inherent capacity to "dissociate": that is, to move between different feeling states and even different aspects of identity. To one degree or another, we all, according to the occasion, "become" different selves—public, private, adult, child, party person, workaholic. When illness threatens to claim all the territory, the mind creatively features another aspect of the self: a "non-illness" identity that puts aside sickness, if only for a while.

Chapter 6: Going Fishing

15. Recent findings in neurobiology suggest that emotion drives our thinking in more ways than we usually acknowledge. Joseph LeDoux, in *The Emotional Brain: The Mysterious Underpinnings of Emotional Life* (New York: Simon & Schuster, 1998), points out that there are many more neuronal projections from the emotion center of the brain, the amygdala, to the thinking region, the neocortex, than the other way around (pp. 284-85). That is, our feelings affect cognition more than our logical minds affect our feelings.

16. "Dissociation"—splitting off parts of the self, featuring other parts—underlies many of the strategies discussed in the book: transforming, forgetting, forgiving, growing. The flexibility of mind that allows one to let go of pain and focus on what is helpful and hopeful is an antidote to the rigid limitations of "self" that illness imposes.

17. For more on "information personality," see Tara Parker-Pope, "You're Sick. Now What? Knowledge Is Power," *New York Times,* September 30, 2008.

18. For more on the adaptive value of forgetting, see Rusiko Bourtchouladze, *Memories Are Made of This: How Memory Works in Humans and Animals,* excerpted in *Cerebrum,* vol. 4, no. 2 (Spring 2002), p. 114.

19. Jane E. Brody, in an article entitled "Cancer as a Disease, Not a Death Sentence" (*New York Times,* June 17, 2008), points out that many cancers, even those that have metastasized, may not be curable but are still eminently treatable. She cites Dr. Michael Fisch of the MD Anderson Cancer Center in Houston, who describes "the hitchhiker model" of treating advanced cancer: "Time is bought by going from point A, the first-line therapy, to point B, the second-line therapy, to point C, the third line of therapy, and so on. The approach can continue indefinitely,

as long as new therapies become available and patients remain well enough to withstand the rigors of treatment." Dr. Fisch adds the caveat that a meaningful life with cancer depends in part on avoiding the attitude that cancer is hopeless.

20. The discussion of Ron Davis (who died in 2008) comes from Karen Barrow, "Armed with Knowledge, Driven to Fight," *New York Times*, September 23, 2008.

21. Jules Lodish used blink technology to type out his response to journalists from the *New York Times* ("Living for Today, Locked in a Paralyzed Body," by John Schwartz and James Estrin, *New York Times*, November 7, 2004).

22. Bauby's *The Diving Bell and the Butterfly* (New York: Vintage International, 1998) was written with the help of assistants who recited the alphabet to him again and again, recording a given letter when he blinked.

Chapter 7: Just My Luck

23. *Lupus* is Latin for "wolf": some early observers thought that the rash looked like the bite of a wolf.

24. In a classic article entitled "The Environment and Disease: Association or Causation?" (*Proceedings of the Royal Society of Medicine*, vol. 58, no. 5 [May 1965], pp. 295–300), Sir Austin Bradford Hill outlines aspects of the association between two variables that might legitimately lead to the assumption of a causal connection: strength of the association, followed by consistency, specificity, temporality, biological gradient, coherence, experiment, and analogy. In the case of temporality, sequence can be an indicator of cause, but Sir Austin points out that sometimes the cart and the horse get reversed. An example: psychosis often follows experimentation with recreational drugs, but, the question has been posed, does pot smoking induce schizophrenia, or does the onset of schizophrenia induce pot smoking?

25. Leslie Snow says she makes it a point to have fun with questionnaires. She refuses to check "yes" on the many items that apply to her, and she's playful on the subject of habits. When her doctor asked her if she drank alcohol every day, she replied, "I try to."

26. "Despite Fear of Diabetes, Many Americans Seen as Continuing Unhealthy Behaviors." Reported on WebMD, March 24, 2009. The survey was conducted by Harris Interactive.

27. Despite the fact that lung cancer is the biggest cancer killer in the U.S., killing more than 160,000 people a year, research on the disease is less well funded than for many other types of cancer, most likely because of

a punitive attitude toward smokers. As Tara Parker-Pope writes in "The Voices of Lung Cancer" on her *New York Times* Well blog of April 22, 2009: "In 2006 the National Cancer Institute spent $1,518 for each new case of lung cancer and $1,630 for each lung cancer death. By comparison, the agency spent $13,452 per death on breast cancer, which takes 41,000 lives annually." Similar social judgments have impeded research on AIDS and HIV.

28. Medical writer Abigail Zuger reports on a diabetic patient whose blood sugars remained sky-high despite diet, insulin, and pills. She took him off a few medications, and at the same time, the patient started going to church. "He never had another elevated blood sugar reading. He was cured. Cured!" "Magnificent Medical Miracles, and Everyday Ones, Too," *New York Times,* November 25, 2008.

Chapter 8: The Growing Point

29. The process of forging permanent neural pathways, whereby changes occur at the synapse between neurons that enhance and strengthen the connection, is called long-term potentiation.

30. New learning is another concept that underlies many of the strategies outlined in this book. Deepening one's sense of self, transforming and exploring, overcoming obstacles, and, as we'll see, sharing with others—all these approaches depend on an open mind that seeks connections and takes in new experiences. This sort of openness may seem contrary to the dissociative process described elsewhere, which would seem to be more about splitting off and forgetting than about integrating and absorbing. The truth is, you need everything you've got—all aspects of yourself and all the mental capacities available to you—to live well with chronic illness. Depending on the circumstances, sometimes it's good to open up, and sometimes it's necessary to shut down. Sometimes it's possible to feel whole and integrated, and sometimes different facets of the self emerge. The people who are most resilient tend to use the whole toolbox.

31. Openness and playfulness are helpful in negotiating a long illness. People who have a sense of humor—which is another way of saying "an open mind"—are often noticeably resilient. They can entertain more than one possibility (or, to put it another way, access more than one neural network), which helps them move beyond rigid and confining positions.

Chapter 9: Caretaking

32. For a discussion of the effects of chronic illness on families, see Susan McDaniel, Jeri Hepworth, and William J. Doherty, *Medical Family Therapy: A Biopsychosocial Approach to Families with Health Problems* (New York: Basic Books, 1992), pp. 192–93.
33. The John Donne quote is from the poem "A Nocturnal upon St. Lucy's Day, Being the Shortest Day": "The general balm th' hydroptic earth hath drunk, / Whither, as to the bed's-feet, life is shrunk."